OXFORD MEDICAL PUBLICATIONS

Colour Atlas of
Paediatric Haematology

THIRD EDITION

Colour Atlas of Paediatric Haematology

Third Edition

Ian M. Hann

Department of Haematology and Oncology,
Great Ormond Street Hospital for Children NHS Trust,
Great Ormond Street, London

Brian D. Lake

Professor of Histochemistry,
Great Ormond Street Hospital for Children NHS Trust,
Great Ormond Street, London

John Lilleyman

Professor of Paediatric Oncology,
St Bartholomew's Hospital Medical College, London

and

Jon Pritchard

Department of Haematology and Oncology,
Great Ormond Street Hospital for Children NHS Trust,
Great Ormond Street, London

Oxford   New York   Toronto
OXFORD UNIVERSITY PRESS
1996

Oxford University Press, Walton Street, Oxford OX2 6DP

Oxford New York
Athens Auckland Bangkok Bombay
Calcutta Cape Town Dar es Salaam Delhi
Florence Hong Kong Istanbul Karachi
Kuala Lumpur Madras Madrid Melbourne
Mexico City Nairobi Paris Singapore
Taipei Tokyo Toronto
and associated companies in
Berlin Ibadan

Oxford is a trade mark of Oxford University Press

Published in the United States
by Oxford University Press Inc., New York

First edition published 1983
Second edition published 1990
Third edition published 1996

A catalogue record for this book is available from the British Library

Library of Congress Cataloging in Publication Data
Colour atlas of paediatric haematology / Ian M. Hann . . . [et al.} – 3rd ed.
(Oxford medical publications)
Includes bibliographical references and index.
1. Pediatric hematology—Atlases. I. Hann, Ian M. II. Series.
[DNLM: 1. Hematologic Diseases—in infancy & childhood—atlases.
WS 17 C719 1996]
RJ411.C64 1966   618.92'15—dc20   95-21319
ISBN 0-19-262696-5

Typeset by Cotswold Typesetting Ltd, Gloucester
Printed and bound in Hong Kong

Foreword

by
David Weatherall

Regius Professor of Medicine,
University of Oxford

There must be few 'adult haematologists' who have not gazed in gloomy despair at a blood film from a newborn infant and speculated uneasily on whether the bizarre morphological changes of the red cells are within normal limits. Certainly, I have spent a few sleepless nights over wild white cell changes in the blood of young children with viral illnesses, wondering if I was seeing an unusual form of leukaemia or whether it is just a reflection of the perversity of childhood to react to infection in this way. Indeed, it is sobering to reflect that the majority of haematologists who look at blood films or bone marrows of infants or young children have had little or no training in paediatrics. In many countries, and Great Britain is no exception, paediatric haematology is the Cinderella of the paediatric sub-specialties. Most paediatricians, like general physicians, are unable to find their way round a blood film or marrow and are totally reliant on their laboratory colleagues, often only experienced in adult blood diseases, for assessing the significance of the haematological findings in sick children. For this reason the authors of this atlas have done a particularly valuable job in bringing together a representative series of pictures of the blood and marrow, both from normal infants and children and from those with haematological disorders peculiar to childhood. I imagine that this book will become a constant companion to haematologists who are called on occasionally to look at the blood or marrow of sick children. At least they will be reassured to see that laboratory artefacts seem to be the same in adult and paediatric practice.

The scope of paediatric haematology has increased immensely over the last few years. It is now possible to obtain blood samples early in fetal life, many new genetic disorders of the blood cells have been defined, the sub-classification of the acute leukaemias has assumed importance in both prognosis and treatment, and a frighteningly complex series of storage disorders have been identified, many of which may present for the first time to the haematologist. With the rapid movement of people round the world paediatric haematologists are often presented with bizarre parasites in the blood, and genetic diseases like the haemoglobinopathies, which used to be so rare in North European countries, are now being seen with increasing frequency in immigrant populations. All these new developments are reflected in this splendid new edition of the *Atlas*.

Paediatric haematology has made a major contribution to the more fundamental aspects of haematological research over the last few years. While in the age of monoclonal antibodies and DNA sequencing it might seem rather old-hat to produce a new atlas of blood morphology, it should be remembered that the application of these new and highly sophisticated techniques is useless unless there has been an accurate morphological diagnosis of the condition being studied. Hence I suspect that this book will also find its way into departments who are working on fundamental haematological research.

Apart from being an acute reminder of increasing age, it is a particular pleasure to be invited to write a foreword to a book in which two of the authors are one's former research fellows or house staff; those involved in medical education need constantly reassuring that it is very difficult permanently to damage the young. I am certain that this atlas will continue to fill an important gap for clinicians and research workers in both developed and developing countries and I wish this new edition as much success as the previous editions.

Preface to the third edition

This volume differs considerably from its predecessor. We have updated disease classifications, added new ones where necessary, and have rewritten many of the remaining 'legends'; we have added new Figures of rare disorders, not previously included in the *Atlas*; and have included new techniques for diagnosis, especially fluorescence *in situ* hybridization which now plays an important part in the accurate diagnoses of childhood tumours including leukaemia. In future (FISH) will probably also be applied to the diagnosis of non-malignant genetic disorders. We have deleted several figures that, in retrospect, made little or no contribution and in one or two cases might be misleading.

We are grateful to the many colleagues who made suggestions for improving the *Atlas*. We hope they will be reasonably satisfied with the outcome!

London and Sheffield   I.M.H
July 1995   B.D.L.
                                                                                J.L.
                                                                                J.P.

Acknowledgements

The production of an atlas such as this could not be done without the begging, borrowing, or perhaps even stealing of slides or transparencies from many sources. We have also received helpful comments on the earlier edition. We are, as a result of the generous donations of slides and of helpful comments, very grateful to the following colleagues both within Great Ormond Street Hospital for Children and from other institutions:- Professor Judith Chessells, Dr Jane Evans, Dr Marian Malone, Dr Owen Smith, Professor Tim Eden, Professor A. V. Hoffbrand, Dr Brenda Gibson, Dr Bernadette Modell, Dr Elizabeth Letsky, Dr David Evans, Dr Sally Davies, Dr R. Goudsmit, Professor Ralph Hendrickse, Dr Ken Clark, Dr M. C. Galvin, Dr Clare Taylor, Dr Raul C. Ribeiro, Dr Silvia Brandalise, Dr Harry Smith, Professor Sinasi Ozsoylu, Mrs Lesley Bloom BSc FIBMS, Miss Julie Cameron FIBMS, and Mr David Wheeler FIBMS MIBiol. We are especially grateful to Mr Rod Hinchliffe FIBMS for his invaluable assistance with Chapter 18. If we have inadvertently omitted anybody, please accept our apologies.

*This book is dedicated to the
staff at Great Ormond Street
and Sheffield Children's Hospital
and also to Julie,
Rebecca
Abigail
&
Jessamy*

Contents

Abbreviations

AHG	anti haemophilic globulin
ALL	acute lymphoblastic leukaemia
AML	acute myeloblastic leukaemia
ANA	antinuclear antibody
C-ALL	common acute lymphoblastic leukaemia
CDA	congenital dyserythropoietic anaemia
CGL	chronic granulocytic leukaemia
CMV	cytomegalovirus
CNS	central nervous system
CSF	cerebrospinal fluid
DIC	disseminated intravascular coagulation
DNA	deoxyribonucleic acid
EB	Epstein–Barr (virus)
EDTA	ethylenediaminetetraacetic acid (anticoagulant)
HE	haematoxylin and eosin (stain)
Hb	haemoglobin
Hb F	fetal haemoglobin
Hb H	haemoglobin H
HDN	haemolytic disease of the newborn
HEMPAS	hereditary erythroblast multinuclearity with positive acid serum lysis test (CDA type II)
HPFH	hereditary persistent fetal haemoglobin
ITP	idiopathic thrombocytopenic purpurea
LE	lupus erythematosus
MCH	mean corpuscular haemoglobin
MCHC	mean corpuscular haemoglobin concentration
MCV	mean cell volume
MGG	May–Grünwald–Giemsa (stain)*
MPS	mucopolysaccharidosis
NAP	neutrophil alkaline phosphatase
NBT	nitro blue tetrazolium
PAS	periodic acid Schiff (stain)
RAEB	refractory anaemia with excess of blasts
RAEB(T)	refractory anaemia with excess of blasts in transformation
T-ALL	acute leukaemia derived from T-lymphoblasts
VMA	vanilylmandelic acid

* Staining is with MGG unless otherwise stated. Details of magnification have only been included where they are of real importance.

1
Normal appearances

The blood

1.1   Cord blood
Blood

Red cells are larger than in later life (MCV 107 fl), and the haemoglobin concentration is greater (mean 16.8 g/dl). Occasional nucleated red cells are seen at birth, but should disappear in a day or two.

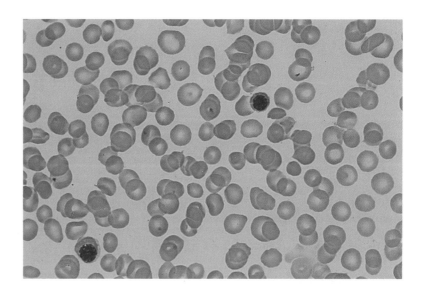

1.2   Band or stab cell
Blood

This cell is the intermediate precursor of the mature polymorph—neutrophil in this instance. The nucleus is crescentic rather than lobed.

These early forms are seen in increased numbers in the blood in response to infection, and estimating their numbers as a ratio to the total white cell count is sometimes used in neonates to help identify those with bacterial infections.

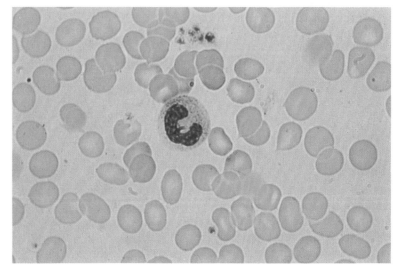

1.3 Neutrophil polymorph
Blood

The mature granulocyte usually has a
three- to four-lobed nucleus. The nuclear
chromatin is clumped and there are no
nucleoli. Nuclear lobes are reduced in
infection (shift to the left) and the
Pelger–Hüet anomaly. Increased
lobulation is present in megaloblastic
anaemia.

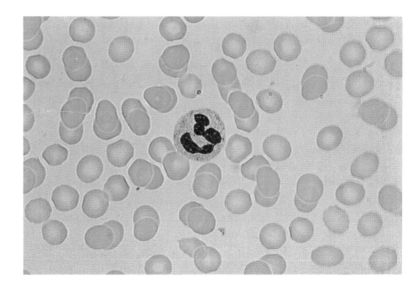

1.4 Eosinophil
Blood

Eosinophils have orange granules on
Romanowsky stains. Typically they are
bilobed. They do not normally exceed
0.4×10^9/l. They are increased in allergy,
atopy, in response to invasive parasites,
drugs, and Hodgkin's disease. Rare
primary eosinophilias occur, both benign
and malignant.

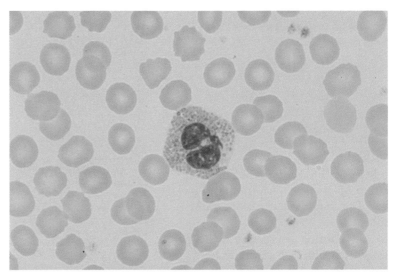

1.5 Basophil
Blood

Basophils are the least common
granulocytes and do not normally exceed
0.1×10^9/l. They are easily recognized.
They may be elevated in hypothyroidism
or chicken pox, but are most commonly
seen in increased numbers in
myeloproliferative disorders.

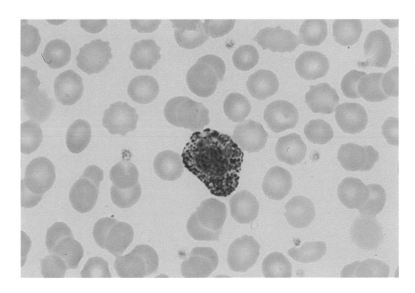

1.6 Monocytes
Blood

Monocytes are derived from a precursor cell common to granulocytes. They typically have irregular nuclei and pale blue cytoplasm on Romanowsky staining. They do not normally exceed $0.8 \times 10^9/l$. Vacuoles and a few azurophil granules are sometimes evident. They increase in some chronic bacterial infections, infestations, virus infections, and autoimmune inflammatory disorders.

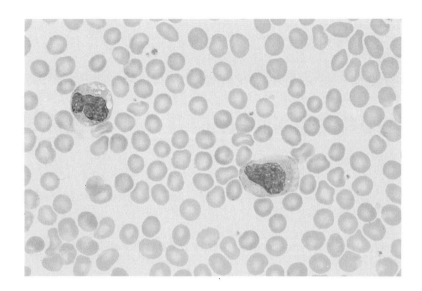

1.7 Mature small lymphocyte
Blood

A normal small, mature lymphocyte with scanty cytoplasm is shown. The blood lymphocyte count varies with age (see section on normal values) and may also be increased in infections (see Chapter 5, on disorders of lymphocytes).

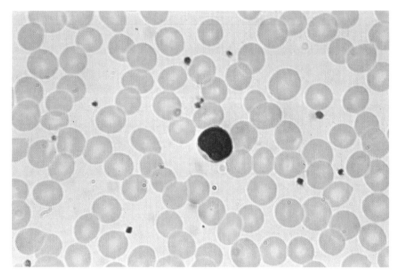

1.8 Mature large lymphocyte
Blood

A variable proportion of normal mature lymphocytes show more cytoplasm which is less basophilic, and the whole cell appears larger.

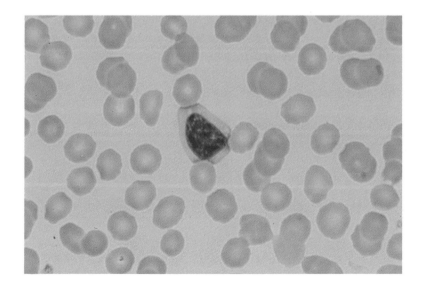

1.9 Large granular lymphocyte
Blood

A variant of the large lymphocyte has fine azurophil granules in the cytoplasm. Such cells frequently show the immunological characteristics of NK (natural killer) lymphocytes.

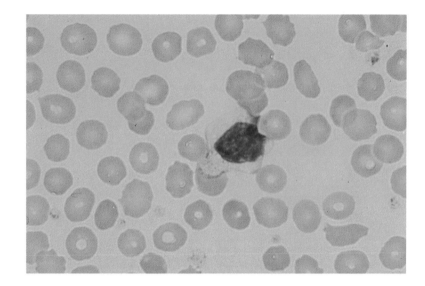

1.10 Plasma cell
Blood film

Plasma cells only rarely circulate in children's blood. They are occasionally seen, usually in response to infection.

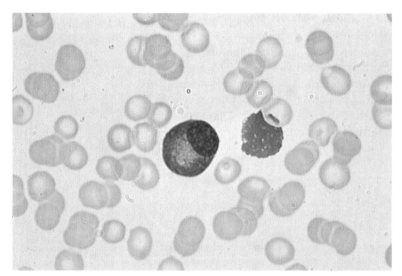

The bone marrow

1.11 Early pronormoblast (arrow)
Bone marrow

This plate shows a large basophilic normoblast. Nucleoli are present. The cytoplasm is intensely basophilic because of its high RNA content.

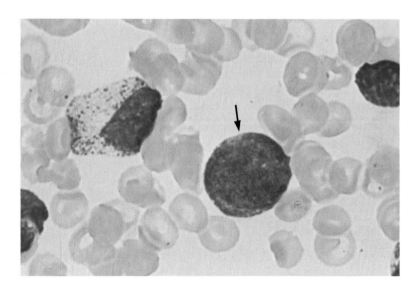

1.12   Early basophilic normoblast
(arrow)
Bone marrow

This cell has slightly less RNA than 1.11 so the basophilia is less intense. Haemoglobin synthesis has started. A myelocyte, a band (stab) cell, and a lymphocyte are also present.

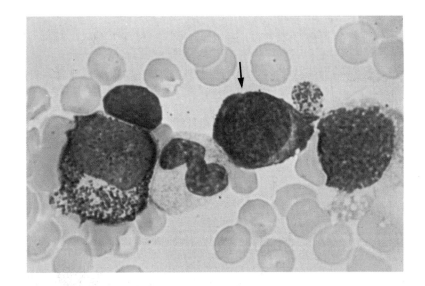

1.13   Developing normoblasts
Bone marrow

This plate shows an intermediate (polychromatic) and a late orthochromatic normoblast. The polychromasia of the intermediate normoblast (below) is a result of its lesser RNA and greater haemoglobin content than that of earlier forms. The orthochromia in the later cell (above) is the result of its increasing haemoglobin content so that the cell takes up the acidophilic component of the Romanowsky stain.

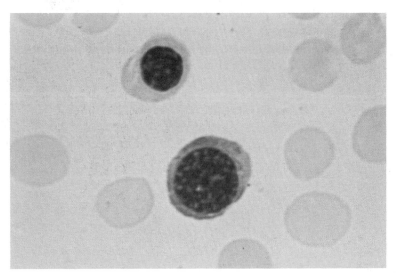

1.14   Late normoblast
Bone marrow

This small well haemoglobinized normoblast (arrowed) and another cell with disintegrating nucleus represent the last stages of normoblast development. A myelocyte is also present.

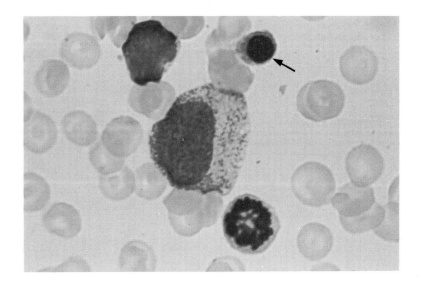

1.15   Promyelocyte
Bone marrow

This is the first differentiated form of developing granulocytes. Nucleoli are visible and most of the granules are the primary azurophilic type, staining red. Some 1 per cent of normal marrow cells are promyelocytes.

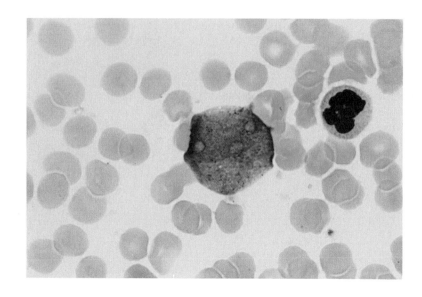

1.16   Developing granulocytes (1)
Bone marrow

Four stages of maturation can be seen in the frame; promyelocyte (pm), myelocyte (m), metamyelocyte (mm), and mature neutrophil (n). Two erythroblasts (eb) are also present.

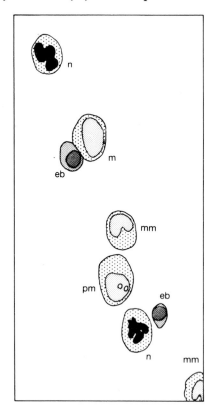

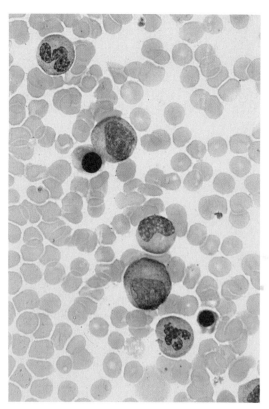

1.17 Developing granulocytes (2)
Bone marrow

Further variants of maturing granulocytes identified as in 1.16.

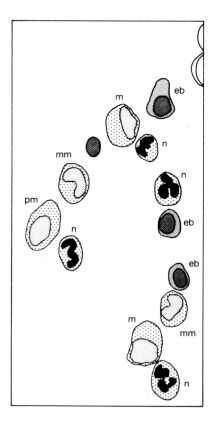
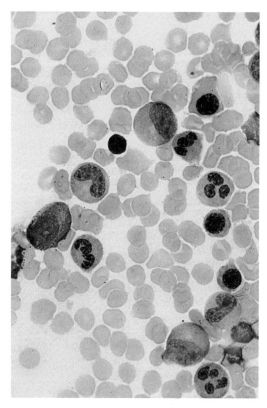

1.18 Megakaryocyte
Blood marrow

This is a mature megakaryocyte showing abundant granular cytoplasm and multiple nuclei. Platelets are produced by a process of 'budding off' the cell, not by mitosis.

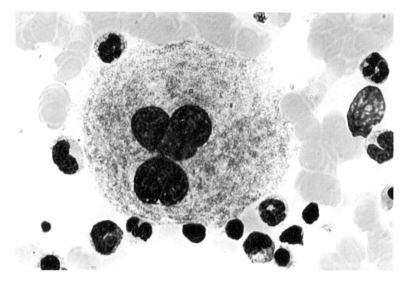

1.19   Normal iron stores
Bone marrow fragments; Perls' iron stain

Iron stores are stained blue and are contained within macrophages.

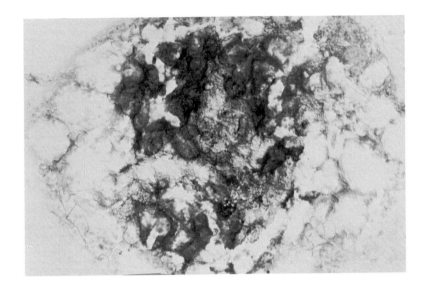

1.20   Macrophage
Bone marrow

Occasional macrophages are seen in the marrows of children who do not have any evidence of a histiocytic syndrome (see Chapter 10) or storage disorder (see Chapter 16). They may show active phagocytosis, and are not necessarily indicative of disease.

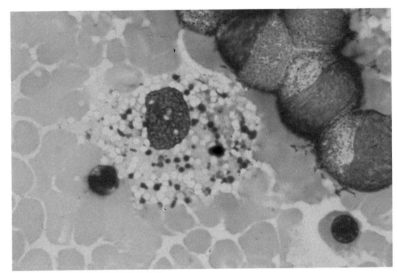

1.21   Osteoblasts
Bone marrow

These large mononuclear cells may be mistaken for tumour cells. They are more frequently encountered in children as marrow may easily be aspirated near an advancing zone of ossification.

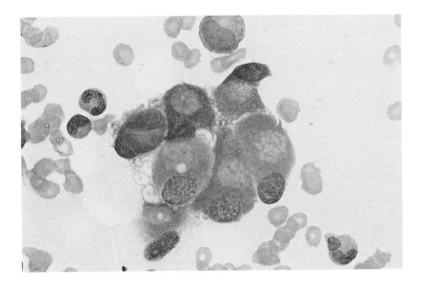

1.22 Osteoclast
Bone marrow

A large multinucleate cell which can be mistaken for an atypical megakaryocyte or a malignant syncytium.

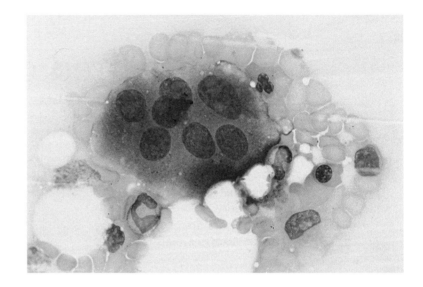

1.23 Normal marrow histology
Trephine biopsy

Overall cellularity varies, but tends to be greater in children. In infancy, fat spaces may be reduced to the point when normality may be mistaken for a myeloproliferative state. This section is from a healthy 4-month-old infant.

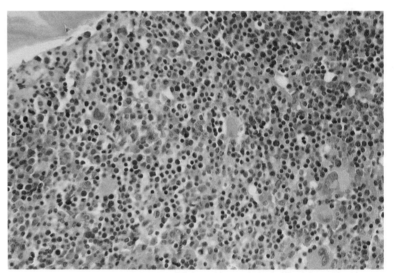

1.24 Normal marrow histology
Trephine biopsy

As 1.23 but from a normal 4-year-old child, to show variable cellularity.

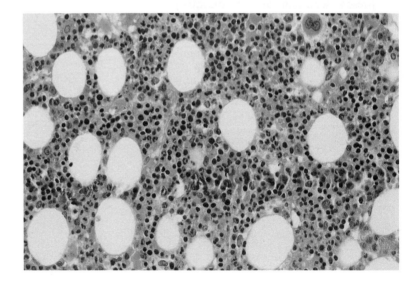

2
Congenital red cell disorders

2.1 Hereditary spherocytosis
Blood film

Blood film from a 6-year-old boy
presenting with jaundice and anaemia. His
mother had a similar history.

Numerous microspherocytes are
present. The larger reticuloctyes are also
seen.

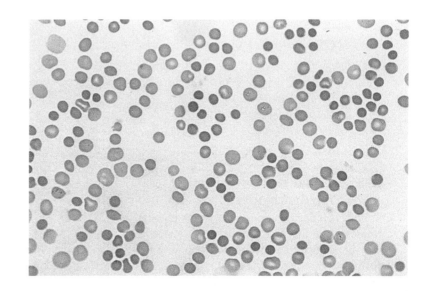

2.2 Hereditary haemolytic elliptocytosis
Blood film

This shows marked poikilocytosis with
bizarre red cell shapes, fragmentation,
micro-ovalocytes, and occasional
spherocytes. An occasional typical
elliptocyte may be seen. Between 10 and
15 per cent of patients with elliptocytosis
present with clinical and laboratory
evidence of haemolysis.

This patient was aged 18 months and
had presented with neonatal jaundice. An
erroneous diagnosis of 'infantile
pyknocytosis' was made. His father had a
similar blood picture.

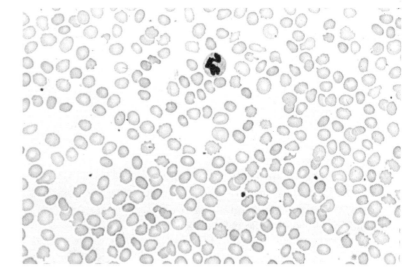

2.3 Hereditary elliptocytosis
Blood film

A majority of the red cells are elliptical in shape but there is no polychromasia. The patient inherited this autosomal dominant condition from his father but neither had evidence of haemolysis.

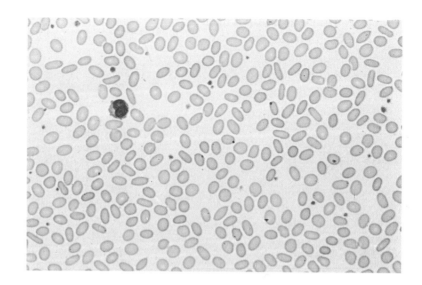

2.4 Hereditary elliptocytosis. Post splenectomy
Blood film

A Howell–Jolly body is seen in the centre of the field, along with other post-splenectomy changes e.g. polychromatic macrocytes, on a background of elliptocytosis.

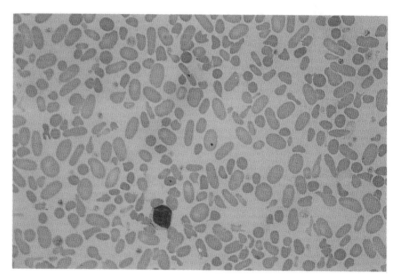

2.5 Hereditary stomatocytosis
Blood film

These red cells, with a central slit-like pale area, are typical of this condition. The same red cell appearances can be acquired in patients on intravenous feeding, with liver disease, or with a red cell sodium pump defect.

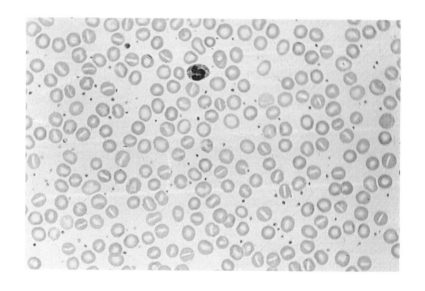

2.6 Hereditary stomatocytosis
Blood; high power

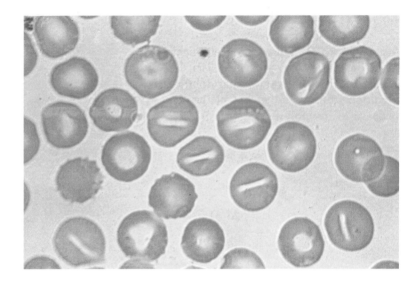

2.7 A-β-lipoproteinaemia
Blood film

This plate shows many 'spur cells' (acanthocytes). These cells can also be seen in liver disease, after splenectomy, and with certain malabsorption syndromes. Coarser 'burr cells' are seen in acute renal failure.

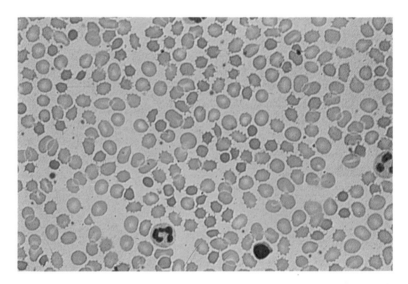

2.8 Hereditary pyropoikilocytosis
Blood film

The illustration shows extreme poikilocytosis with fragments, spherocytes, elliptocytes, 'triangulocytes', and other bizarre red cell forms. Macrocytes (reticulocytes) indicate the continuing severe chronic haemolytic process characteristic of this very rare disorder. The red cells are, as the name implies, sensitive to heat, their membranes 'fragmenting' at 45–46 °C. Transfusion dependency is common but there is frequently a favourable response to splenectomy. The differential diagnosis of this blood film is from disseminated intravascular coagulation (in which the platelets would be low) and homozygous hereditary elliptocytosis. Recently a spectrin abnormality has been demonstrated.

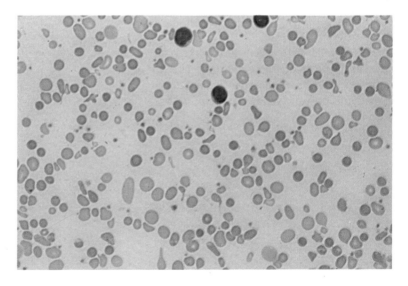

2.9   Pyruvate kinase deficiency
Blood film

Blood film from a 2-year-old presenting with a Hb of 5.0 g/dl and reticulocytes of 30 per cent. In this disorder there is usually only slight anisopoikilocytosis but sometimes an irregularly contracted cell may be seen. This plate shows a 'spicule' or 'Sputnik' cell. In addition, acanthocytes may be seen.

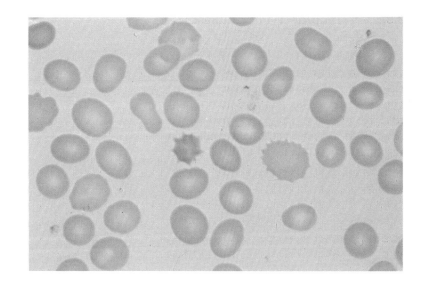

2.10   Favism
Blood film

Several red cells show 'puddling' of their haemoglobin with a residual thin rim of cytoplasm. Some red cell fragmentation and polychromasia are also seen.

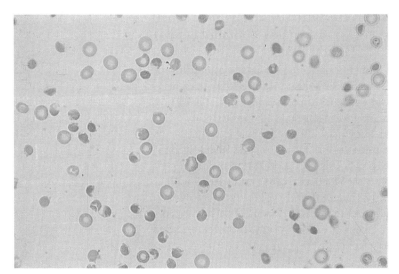

2.11   Triose phosphate isomerase deficiency
Blood film

Deficiency of this glycolytic pathway enzyme is inherited in an autosomal recessive manner. It usually presents with neonatal jaundice. Progressive neurological disorder develops after 6 months of age, along with susceptibility to infection and a muscular disorder with cardiomyopathy.

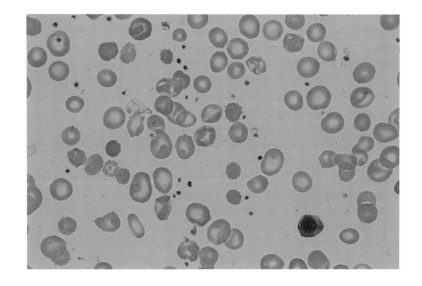

2.12   Pyrimidine-5′-nucleotidase deficiency
Blood film

This shows characteristically prominent basophilic stippling with marked polychromasia. This is a rare autosomal recessive disorder. The patient had a mild haemolytic anaemia with the haemoglobin varying in the range 8–10 g/dl.

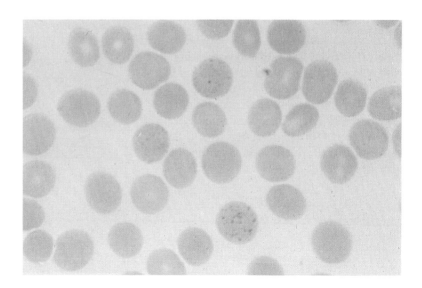

2.13   Hb Bart's Hydrops syndrome (homozygous α′-thalassaemia)
Blood film

Cord blood from a hydropic and stillborn 32-week Singalese infant whose parents both had α′-thalassaemia trait. There are many normoblasts and marked anisocytosis. Hypochromia is only moderate but nearly all the haemoglobin is physiologically non-functional Hb Bart's (70–80 per cent) and Hb H with only traces of embryonic haemoglobins. Hbs A and F are absent. The nucleated red cells are bizarre and binucleate forms are frequent.

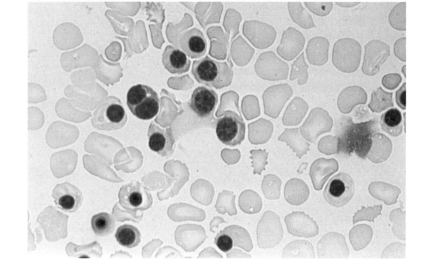

2.14   Hb Bart's Hydrops syndrome
Blood film (see 2.13)

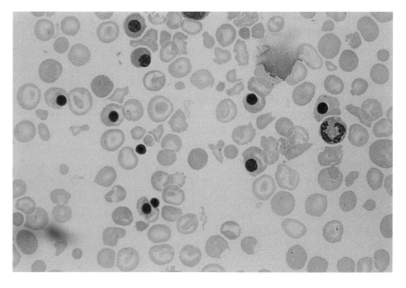

2.15 Hb H disease (α-thalassaemia)
Blood film

This 14-year-old boy has a compensated haemolytic anaemia and moderate splenomegaly. There is marked anisocytosis with many poikilocytes and some target cells. The reticulocyte count is 10–20 per cent. The red cells are hypochromic and microcytic because Hb production is reduced. Hb electrophoresis shows 70–80 per cent Hb A with 10–20 per cent fast-migrating Hb H, normal levels of Hb A_2, and a trace of Hb Bart's. Hb H is unstable (see 2.16).

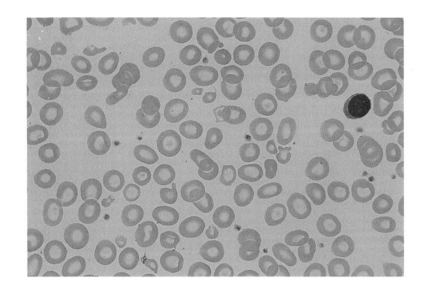

2.16 Hb H preparation
Blood film

In vitro incubation with methyl violet causes precipitation of Hb H as multiple dark-staining spots—a 'golf ball' appearance. (Same patient as 2.15.)

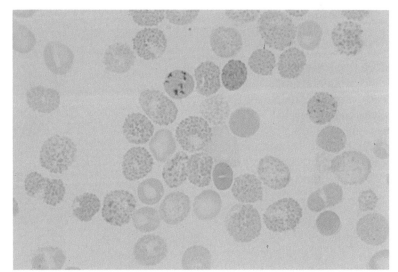

2.17 β-thalassaemia major
Blood film

Blood film from a newly presenting Greek patient. There is marked hypochromia and red cell fragmentation though some normochromic red cells are seen. Nucleated red cells are present. Haemoglobin electrophoresis shows a normal or high-normal Hb A_2 level and up to 95 per cent Hb F. Hb A may be absent (β°-thalassaemia) or present at concentrations in the 2–20 per cent range (β$^+$-thalassaemia). Kleihauer stain shows uneven distribution of Hb F between red cells.

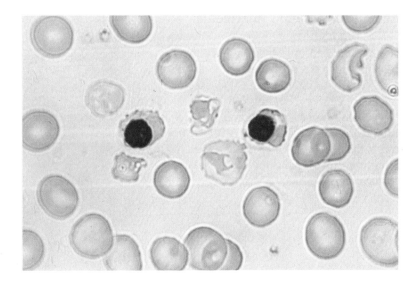

2.18   β-thalassaemia major (untreated)
Blood film

This patient also has folate deficiency. A giant metamyelocyte (see Section 3) is present. Beside it is a dysplastic normoblast showing marked hypochromia. Folate deficiency is secondary to the high red cell turnover resulting from breakdown of inclusion-damaged cells.

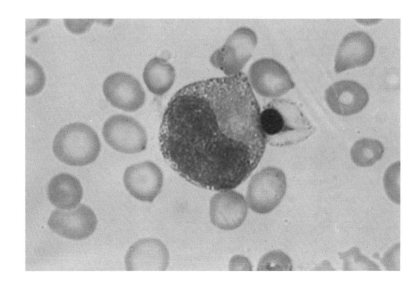

2.19   β-thalassaemia major post-splenectomy
Blood film

More hypochromic red cells are seen. Some contain Howell–Jolly bodies. There is also a giant platelet (see Section 3; post-splenectomy). Methyl violet stain would show many more α-chain inclusions which, prior to splenectomy, would have been 'culled-out' by the spleen.

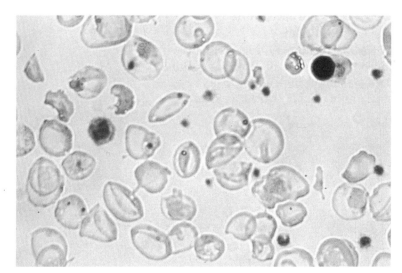

2.20   Thalassaemia intermedia
Blood film

There is marked anisocytosis and hypochromia. No nucleated red cells are seen. Clinically intermediate thalassaemia has many causes including δ-β-thalassaemia homozygosity and interaction of β-thalassaemia with HPFH and α-thalassaemia. Such patients are, by definition, not transfusion dependent but do have chronic haemolysis.

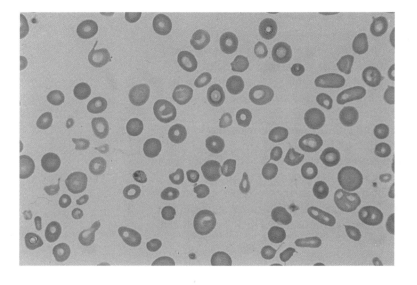

2.21 β-thalassaemia minor (or trait)
Blood film

There is anisocytosis and red cells are microcytic and hypochromic. Target cells and occasional fragmented cells are seen. The major differential diagnosis is iron deficiency. Hb electrophoresis shows increased Hb A_2 (unless there is coexistent iron deficiency) and, in 60–70 per cent of cases, a slightly raised Hb F.

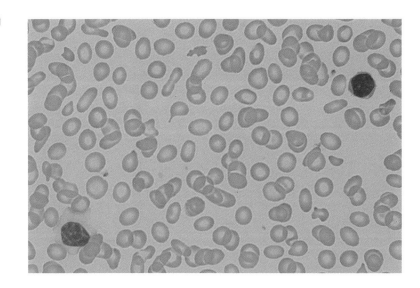

2.22 Homozygous δ-β-thalassaemia
Blood film; Kleihauer stain

This 10-year-old boy had thalassaemia intermedia and Hb electrophoresis showed 100 per cent Hb F. Homozygosity for the HPFH gene was excluded by (a) the child's Arab origin; (b) parental studies; and (c) a demonstration of a marked reduction of γ-compared with α-chain synthesis by his reticulocytes. The apparent heterogeneity of Hb F between red cells is a result of each cell's varying Hb content.

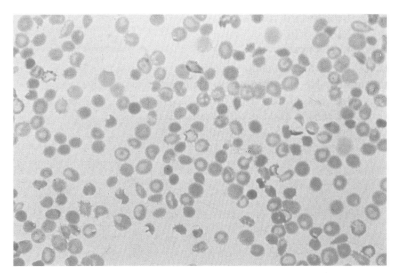

2.23 β-thalassaemia major
Bone marrow

These plates show erythroid hyperplasia and iron-laden macrophages. In 2.23 there are brown siderotic granules, which in 2.24 are confirmed as iron by Perls' stain.

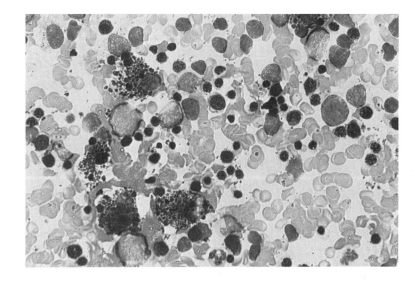

2.24 β-thalassaemia major
Bone marrow; Perls' stain
(see 2.23)

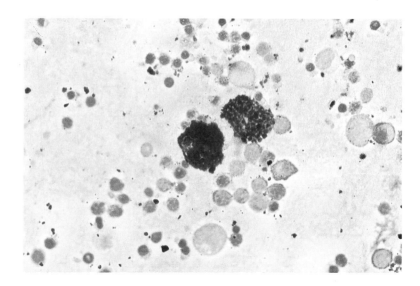

2.25 Sickle-cell anaemia
Blood film

This child—a West Indian aged 10
years—presented with hip pain and
pneumonia. He was in a sickle-cell crisis.
Numerous sickled cells are present. Hb
electrophoresis showed predominant Hb S
with 5 per cent Hb F and a normal Hb A$_2$
level and no Hb A.

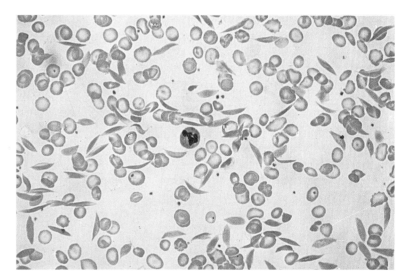

2.26 Sickle-cell anaemia
Blood film

Another patient with sickle cell disease,
showing a more usual pattern with fewer
sickled cells ('drapanocytes') and
prominent target cells.

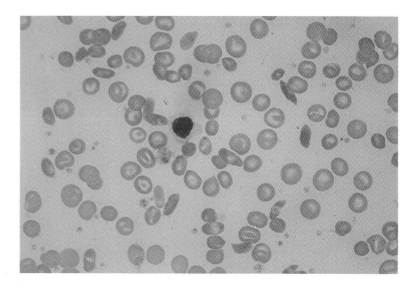

2.27 Sickle beta (Sβ₀) thalassaemia. Blood film

Hypochromic cells, target cells, sickled cells and normoblasts are seen, with features of auto-splenectomy. Haemoglobin electrophoresis shows 0–20 per cent Hb A, 30–40 per cent Hb F, 40–50 per cent Hb S, and normal or increased Hb A$_2$.

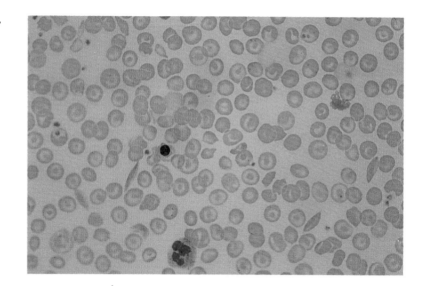

2.28 Sickle β-thalassaemia Blood film

One sickled cell and many target cells are seen. The red cells are hypochromic. Hb electrophoresis shows 0–20 per cent Hb A; 30–40 per cent Hb F; 40–50 per cent Hb S; and normal or increased Hb A$_2$.

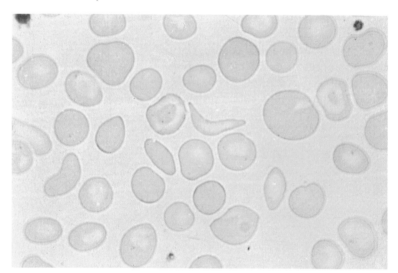

2.29 Haemoglobin S-C disease. Blood film

This is a typical blood film with prominent target cells and infrequent sickled cells.

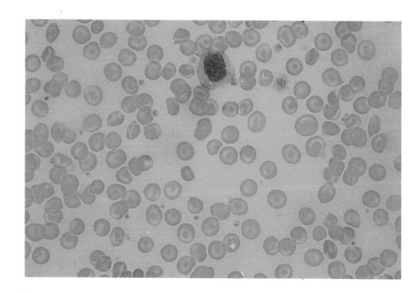

2.30   Haemoglobin C (Hb CC)
Blood film

Target cells are very prominent
in this benign disorder.

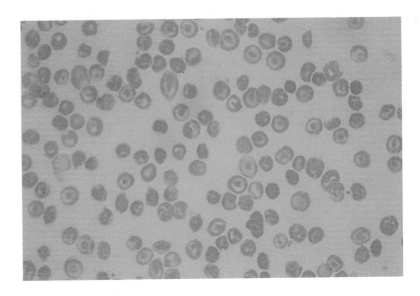

2.31   Hb E trait
Blood film

Blood film from an Indian child. The red
cells are normochromic and target cells
are present; differentiation from Hb C
trait is by the patient's ethnic origin and
by Hb electrophoresis.

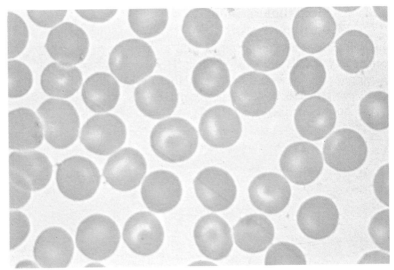

2.32   Hb E-thalassaemia
Blood film

There is marked anisocytosis and
hypochromia. A dysplastic nucleated red
cell is seen in 2.32 and target cells are
frequent. These patients are almost always
transfusion dependent.

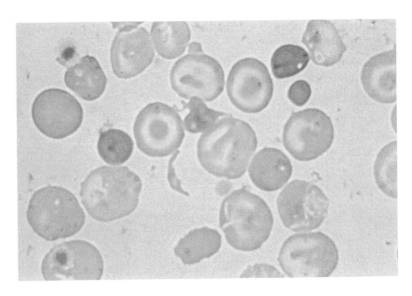

2.33 Hb E-thalassaemia
Blood film. See 2.32

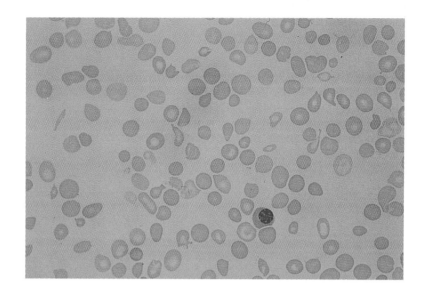

2.34 Unstable haemoglobin (Hb Hammersmith)
Blood film

The MGG film shows a marked anisocytosis with polychromasia. There are poikilocytes and the red cell in the centre of the field has prominent basophilic stippling. There are about 50 unstable variants of Hb. Under stress these Hb's denature easily, precipitate within the cells and form Heinz bodies. These rigid inclusions cause premature red cell destruction in the spleen. The consequent haemolytic anaemia may be severe (Hb Hammersmith or Hb Bristol) or mild to moderate (Hb Köln).

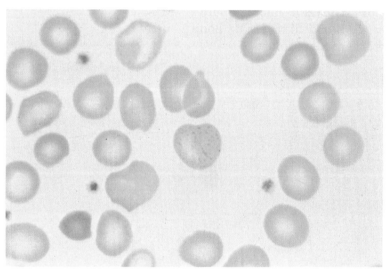

2.35 Haemolytic anaemia due to unstable Hb Köln
Blood film

This is an unstable haemoglobin resulting in a congenital Heinz-body haemolytic anaemia (c.f. 2.36). Affected patients have a congenital non-spherocytic haemolytic anaemia, which in this case is of moderate severity. Splenectomy may be of value and oxidant drugs must be avoided. The blood film shows the presence of basophilic inclusions (arrowed), which in this instance were usually single, although in other cases they are multiple. The red cells are hypochromic with some crenation but spherocytes are usually only present during a haemolytic crisis.

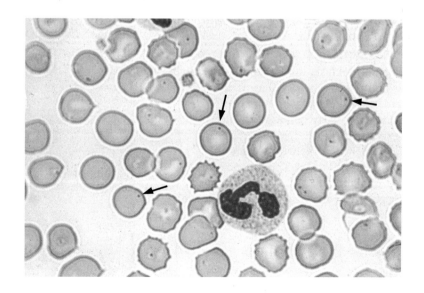

2.36   Unstable haemoglobin
Blood film; Heinz body
preparation

This supravital stain using methyl violet
shows Heinz bodies as dark, round
precipitates in the red cells. The bodies are
attached to the cell membrane. The blood
is from the same patient as in 2.34. Heinz
bodies are more plentiful after
splenectomy.

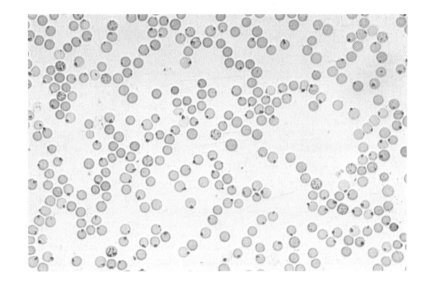

2.37   Unstable haemoglobin
Blood film; Heinz body
preparation

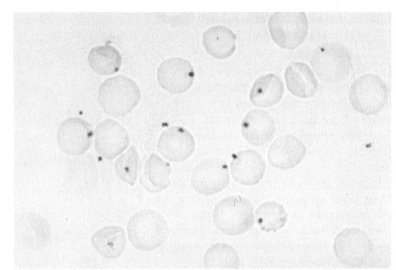

2.38   Congenital erythropoietic
porphyria
Bone marrow (UV fluorescence)

The normoblasts in this condition contain
uroporphyrin 1 which fluoresces intensely
under UV light at 400 nm. The disease
presents in early childhood with
destructive skin lesions in areas exposed
to sunlight and with hirsutism and
hyperpigmentation. The patient's urine is
red or pink. These features have been
suggested as the origin for the 'werewolf'
stories.

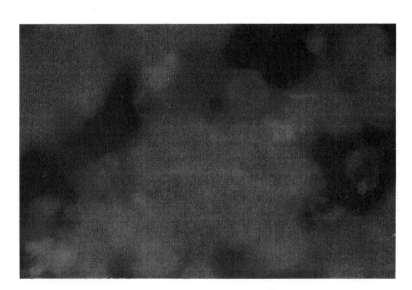

2.39 Diamond–Blackfan syndrome
Bone marrow
Red cell precursors are virtually absent.
Iron-laden macrophages are seen (2.40)
and the iron stain (2.41) shows increased
stores.

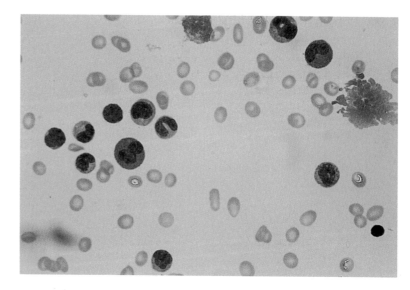

2.40 Diamond–Blackfan syndrome
Bone marrow (see 2.39)
Iron-laden macrophages are present.

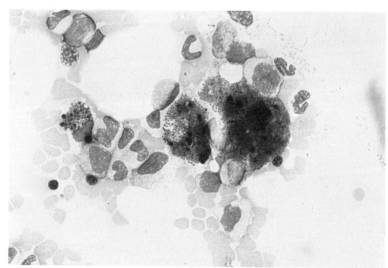

2.41 Diamond–Blackfan syndrome
Bone marrow (Perls' iron stain)

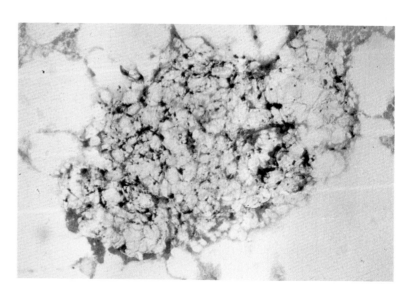

2.42 Congenital dyserythropoietic anaemia (CDA) type I
Blood film

There is marked anisocytosis with polychromasia. 'Helmet cells', 'tadpole cells', and small fragments are seen.

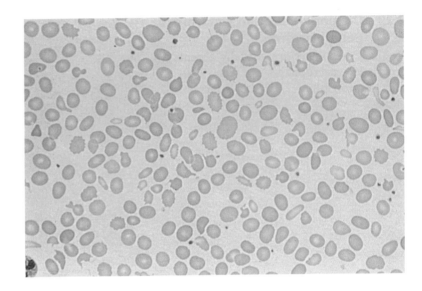

2.43 CDA type I
Blood film. See 2.42

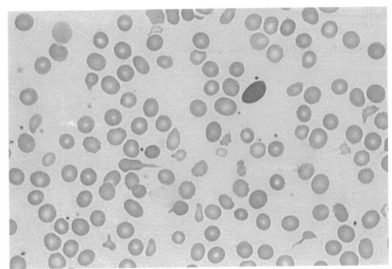

2.44 CDA type I
Blood film

Examples of red cell fragmentation.

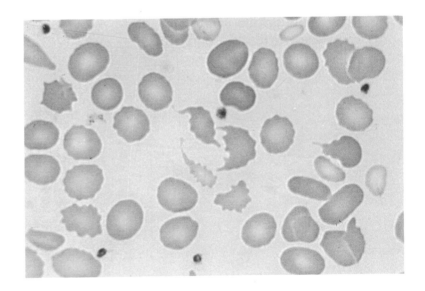

2.45 CDA type I
Blood film
Intense basophilic stippling in a red cell.

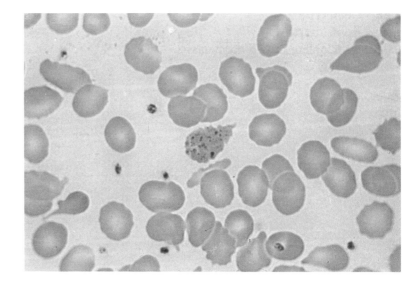

2.46 CDA type I
Bone marrow
All the plates show characteristic erythroid hyperplasia with megaloblastosis and giant metamyelocytes. Diagnostic features are internuclear bridging—a strand of chromatin between two nuclei (2.47, 2.46); basophilic stippling in normoblasts (2.48); and abnormal nuclear pyknosis in normoblasts (2.49). No serological abnormalities are present. The patient presented with anaemia, splenomegaly, and a slightly raised bilirubin. Diagnosis may be delayed until adolescence.

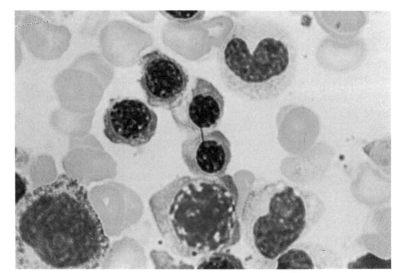

2.47 CDA type I
Bone marrow
Internuclear bridging.

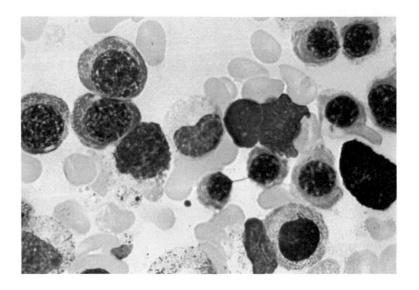

2.48   CDA type I
Bone marrow
Basophilic stippling in two normoblasts.

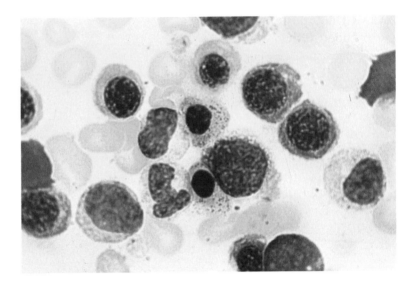

2.49   CDA type I
Bone marrow
A normoblast pyknotic nucleus.

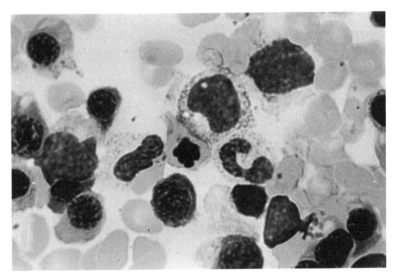

2.50   CDA type II, 'HEMPAS'
Blood film
This shows less anisocytosis and
poikilocytosis than the CDA I blood film.

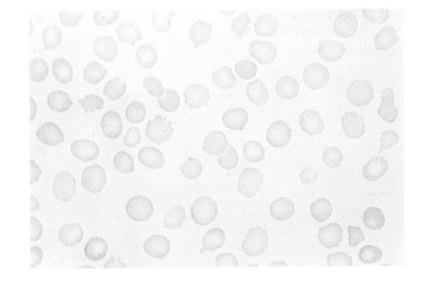

2.51 CDA type II
Bone marrow

This low-power view shows erythroid hyperplasia. Multinuclearity is prominent and present in the late erythroblasts. There are few internuclear bridges. Megaloblastic changes are not as marked as in CDA type I. This is the commonest CDA and is diagnosed by a positive acid serum lysis (Ham's test) as well as by the morphological changes. The patient, aged 8 years, presented with a mild anaemia, mild jaundice, and hepatosplenomegaly. She also had gallstones.

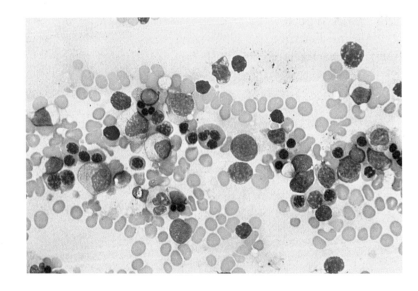

2.52 CDA type II
Bone marrow

High-power views showing in more detail the bizarre appearances of red cell precursors.

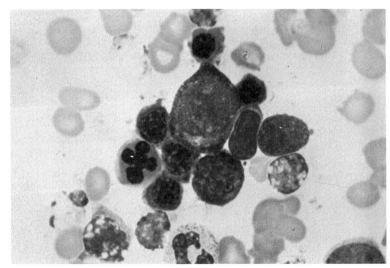

2.53 CDA type II
Bone marrow

Multinucleate red cell precursors.

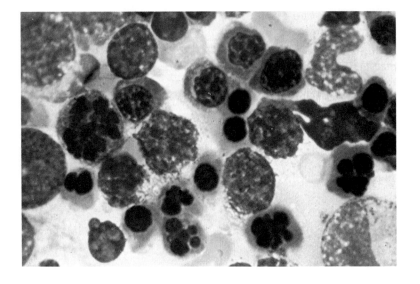

2.54 CDA type II
Bone marrow
Iron-laden macrophage.

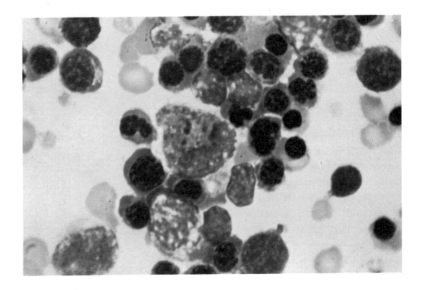

2.55 CDA type II
Bone marrow (see 2.52)

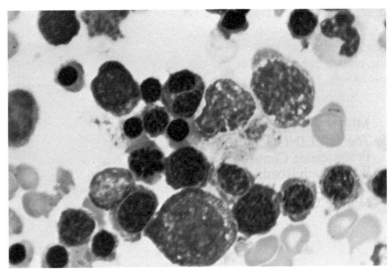

2.56 CDA type III
Blood film
There is marked poikilocytosis, macrocytosis, and polychromasia. This is the rarest form of CDA. Diagnosis may be delayed until adult life and patients present with anaemia. The liver and spleen may be palpable. The gene location has recently been mapped to 15q21–q22 (Lind *et al. (1995) Hum. Mol. Genet.*, **4**, 109).

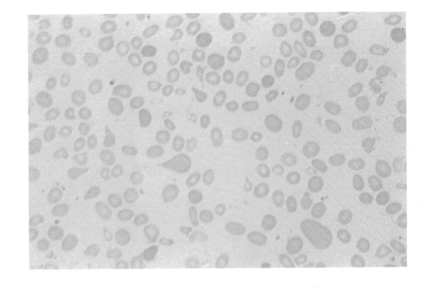

2.57 CDA type III
Blood film
Marked red cell basophilic stippling.

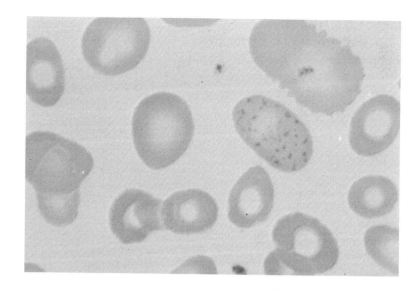

2.58 CDA type III
Bone marrow
This low-power view shows intense erythroid activity with many multinucleate cells. The next three plates show in more detail the multinuclearity, basophilic stippling, and nuclear lobulation. Multinuclearity is sometimes so striking that the cells are called 'gigantoblasts'.

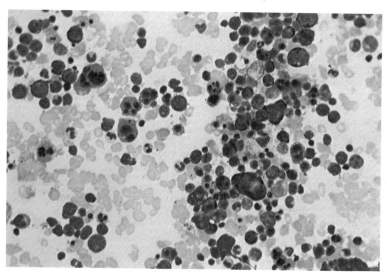

2.59 CDA type III
Bone marrow; high power
Nuclear lobulation and multinucleate cells.

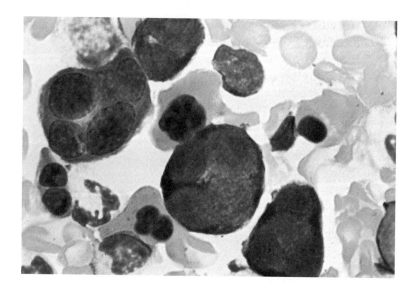

2.60   CDA type III
Bone marrow; high power
Multinuclearity and basophilic stippling.

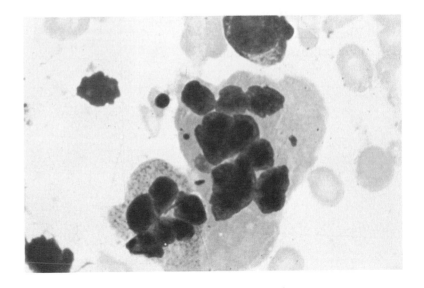

2.61   CDA type III
Bone marrow; high power
'Gigantoblasts' (see 2.58).

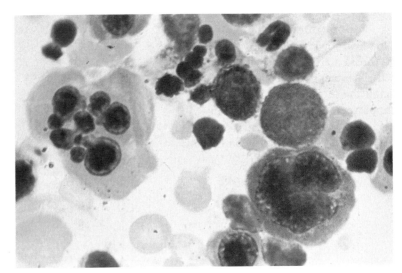

2.62   Hereditary sideroblastic anaemia (post-transfusion)
Blood film
This shows many hypochromic microcytes. The normochromic cells may be residual transfused cells. In 2.63 the marrow shows ring sideroblasts. This is inherited as a sex-linked recessive disorder. The bone marrow is normoblastic.

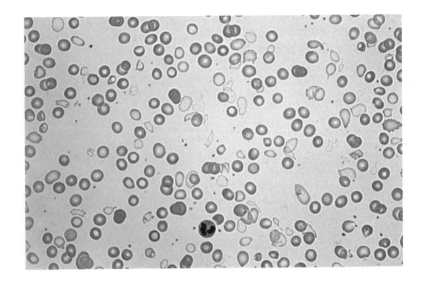

2.63 Hereditary sideroblastic anaemia
Marrow; iron stain
Ring sideroblasts are present in normoblastic marrow.

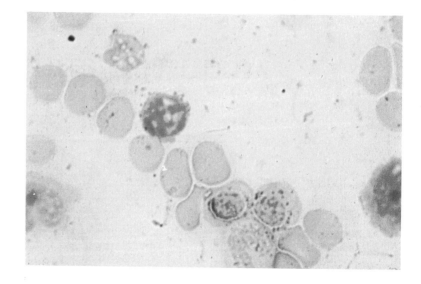

2.64 Fanconi's anaemia—dyserythropoiesis
Bone marrow
Both plates show abnormal red cell precursors—here a 'trefoil' nucleated red cell. The patient was a 2-year-old girl who also had a congenital heart defect and abnormal forearms. She had a normal Hb and white cell count but was thrombocytopenic. She later developed complete marrow aplasia.

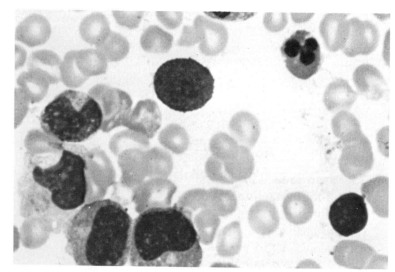

2.65 Fanconi's anaemia
Bone marrow
Abnormal vacuolation of red cell precursors (arrow); this is also said to occur in some cases of chloramphenicol myelotoxicity and Schwachman–Diamond syndrome.

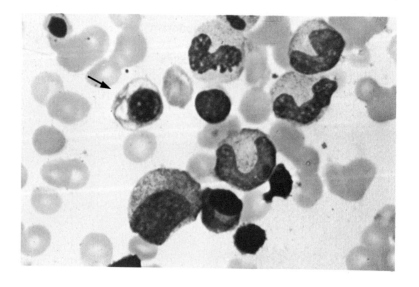

3
Acquired and secondary red cell disorders

3.1 Simple iron lack
Blood

Haemoglobin 6.6 g/dl; MCV 55 fl, MCH 12 pg; gross hypochromia and microcytosis. Haemoglobin A_2 concentration normal. Five-year-old Asian child with gross dietary deficiency, a particular problem for this ethnic group.

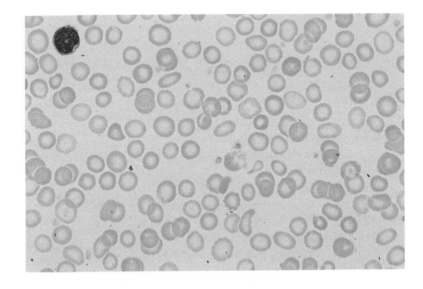

3.2 Iron lack with co-existent β-thalassaemia trait
Blood

Haemoglobin 8.8 g/dl; ferritin 3 μg/l; haemoglobin A_2 5.5 per cent, F 2.6 per cent. Asian child with dietary deficiency. Thalassaemia trait in this ethnic group not infrequently associates with iron deficiency and the two are not mutually exclusive. The haemoglobin A_2 concentration is rarely if ever affected sufficiently by the iron deficiency to become unreliable.

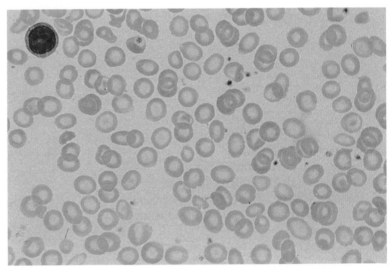

3.3 Iron lack due to bleeding
Blood

Haemoglobin 6.1 g/dl. Asian child returned from Pakistan with heavy infestation of hookworm (Ankylostoma duodenale). The patient also had a striking eosinophilia—1.2×10^9/l.

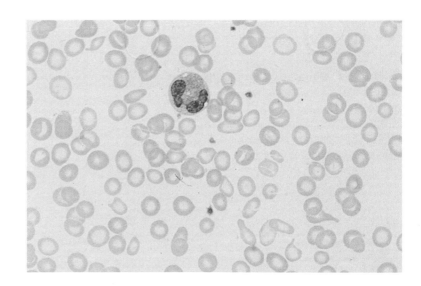

3.4 Partially treated iron lack
Blood

Six days of iron supplements to a starting haemoglobin of 5.4 g/dl; rise of concentration to 6.7 g/dl. Dimorphic picture; note larger polychromatic cells emerging.

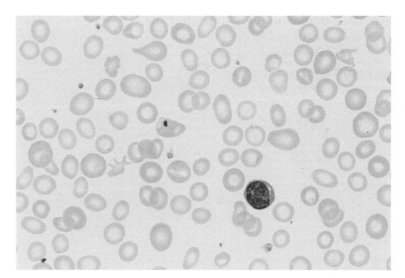

3.5 Megaloblastic anaemia—dietary folate deficiency
Blood

Gross anisocytosis with normochromic oval macrocytes. MCV 102 fl; serum folate 0.2 μg/l; red cell folate 65 μg/l (lower limit of normal 2 and 170 μg respectively). Four-year-old girl, anorexic following cancer chemotherapy.

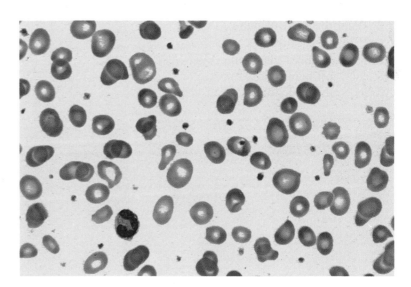

3.6   Megaloblastic anaemia—dietary folate deficiency
Blood

Child of 10 months with strict vegan parents and diet deficient in vitamin B_{12} and folate. Hypersegmented neutrophils of this type are seen in all varieties of macrocytic anaemia that result from megaloblastic haemopoiesis.

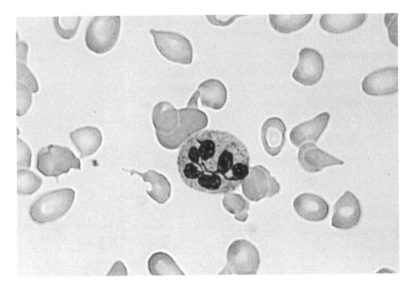

3.7   Megaloblastic anaemia—marrow appearances (red cells)
Bone marrow

Intermediate and late megaloblasts, the latter showing orthochromasia, alongside polychromatic normoblasts. The marrow is from the child illustrated in 3.5.

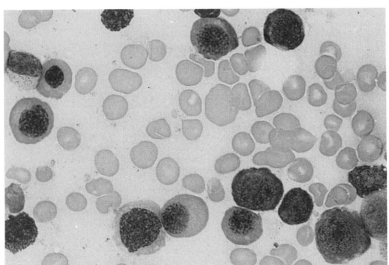

3.8   Pseudomegaloblasts
Bone marrow

Bizarre megaloblast-like erythroblasts seen in a child just completing a course of cytosine arabinoside for acute leukaemia.

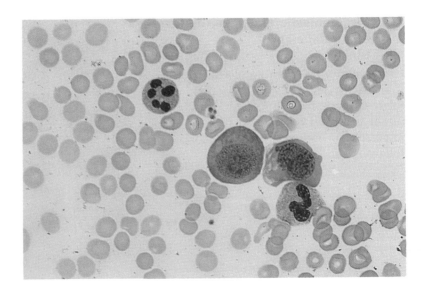

3.9 Megaloblastic anaemia—marrow appearances (white cells)
Bone marrow

Giant myelocytes and metamyelocytes. Note normal small lymphocyte as size marker. A 2-year-old child with congenital deficiency of transcobalamin II.

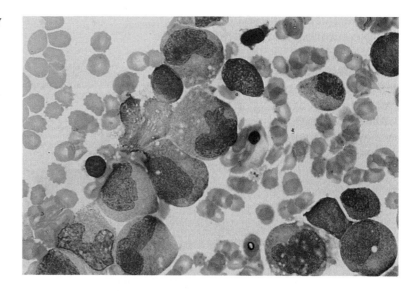

3.10 Megaloblastic anaemia—iron stores
Bone marrow; Perls' stain

Abundant stainable iron in marrow particle seen at lower power.

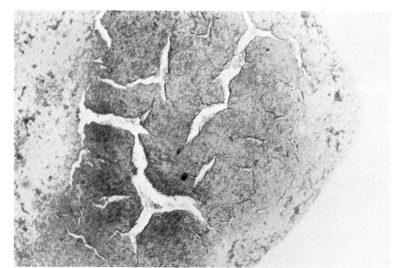

3.11 Megaloblastic anaemia—sideroblasts
Bone marrow; Perls' stain

Normal sideroblast staining is seen in most uncomplicated megaloblastic anaemias (arrowed cells). Ring sideroblasts are not a feature.

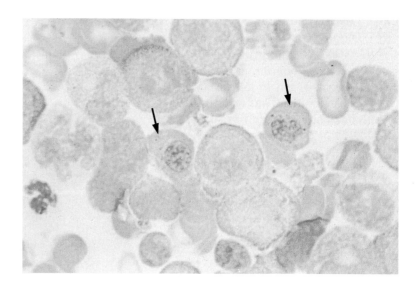

3.12   Megaloblastic anaemia—combined iron and folate deficiency
Bone marrow

Red cell megaloblastic changes are masked to some extent when iron deficiency co-exists, but giant metamyelocytes are still evident. From a child with gluten enteropathy.

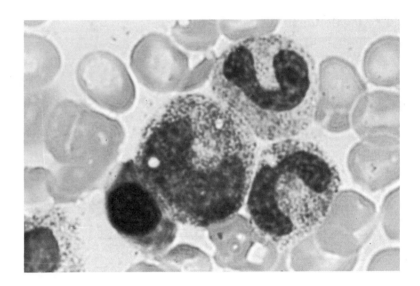

3.13   Coeliac disease
Blood

In addition to features of folate deficiency (hypersegmented neutrophil), this example also shows evidence of associated hyposplenism—fragmented red cells and Howell–Jolly bodies.

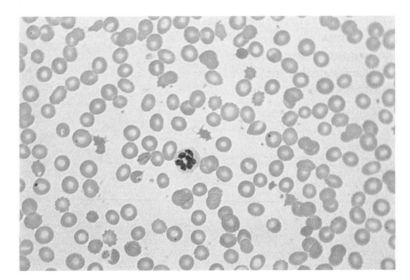

3.14   Lead poisoning
Blood

A red cell with prominent basophilic stippling is seen. Hypochromia was not particularly prominent in this instance. The 2-year-old patient was investigated for anaemia and colic. He was seen to nibble at paint on a window frame.

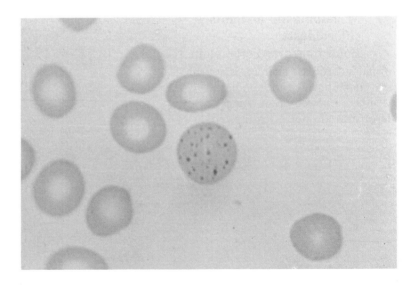

3.15 Chronic renal failure
Blood

Haemoglobin 5.2 g/dl; normochromic and unremarkable red cells. Creatinine 1085 μmol/l; urea 49.2 mmol/l; MCV 83 fl; MCH 25.5; reticulocytopenia. Thirteen-year-old boy with obstructive uropathy at 6 months leading to nephrectomy on one side and a poorly functioning kidney on the other; undialysed.

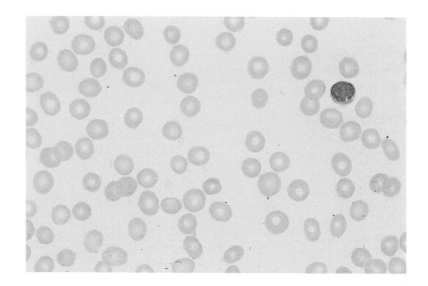

3.16 Chronic renal failure
Blood

Seven-year-old child with congenital dysplastic kidneys on long-term peritoneal dialysis. Haemoglobin 8.8 g/dl; MCV 90 ft; MCH 30.9 (untransfused). Minimal macrocytosis; red cells unremarkable.

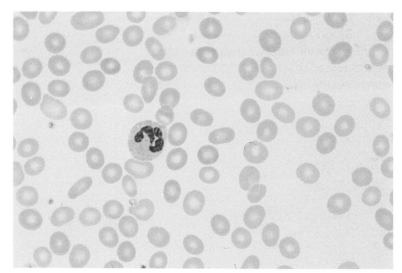

3.17 Liver disease—sepsis and intravascular coagulation
Blood

Terminal hepatic failure in a child of 7 months with associated sepsis and intravascular coagulation. Bilirubin 52 μmol/l; ALT 423 u/l. Target cells, crenated cells, and irregularly contracted cells.

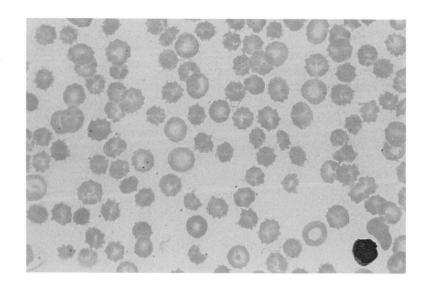

3.18   Liver disease—biliary atresia
Blood

Biliary atresia in a five-year-old. Well, with progressive obstructive jaundice awaiting liver transplantation. Bilirubin 185 μmol/l; ALT 76 u/l; alkaline phosphatase 1206 u/l.

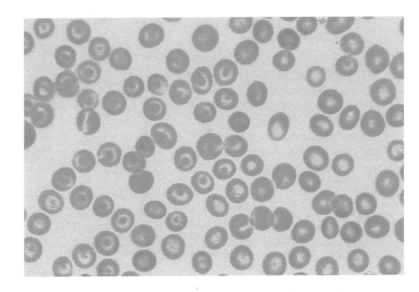

3.19   Liver disease—biliary atresia
Blood

A further case of biliary atresia with more marked red cell changes—target cells, leptocytes (thin cells).

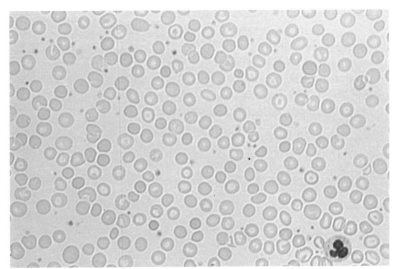

3.20   Liver disease—trauma
Blood

Five-year-old with massive laceration of the liver. Shows spherocytes, fragmented cells, and spiculated cells.

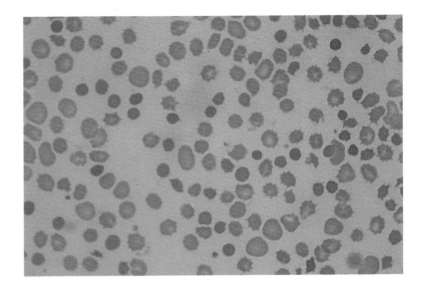

3.21 Transient erythroblastopenia of childhood
Blood

Profound normochromic anaemia with absent or grossly reduced reticulocytes in an otherwise well child. Often there is an associated thrombocytosis. White cells are unremarkable. The cause is not clear—it is not usually associated with parvovirus infection.

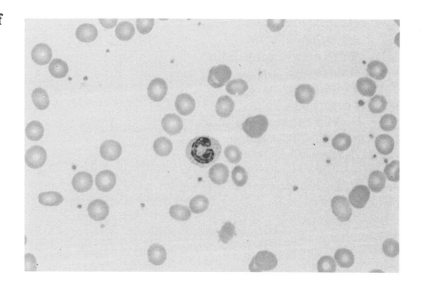

3.22 Transient erythroblastopenia of childhood
Bone marrow

Absent or grossly reduced erythroblasts. Granulopoiesis is unremarkable. The relative (or occasionally absolute) lymphocytosis can give rise to an erroneous diagnosis of lymphoblastic leukaemia.

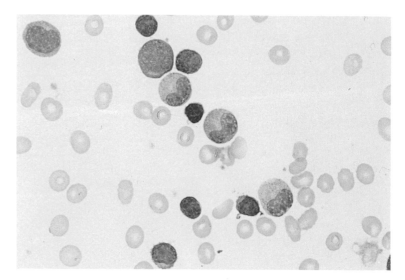

3.23 Acquired haemolytic anaemia— immune warm type
Blood

Male infant aged two with idiopathic warm autoimmune haemolytic anaemia. Antibody auto-pan with no red cell antigen specificity. Hb 6.1 g/dl, MCV 108 fl, reticulocytes 980×10^9/l. Some cell debris and clumping.

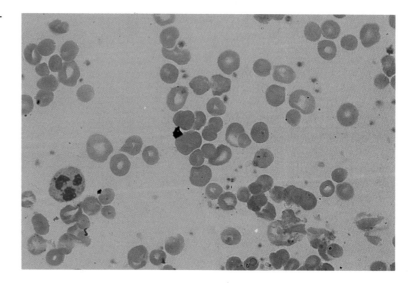

3.24 Haemolytic anaemia— reticulocyte stain
Reticulocyte preparation

Red cells incubated with supravital stain (brilliant cresyl blue). Young ones with residual RNA take up the stain and show a reticular pattern. Normally there are fewer than $100 \times 10^9/l$, but their numbers greatly increase in haemolytic anaemias of any cause—provided marrow function is normal. They also increase in response to blood loss.

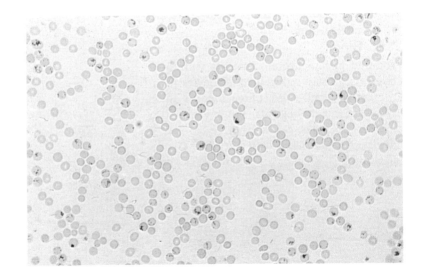

3.25 Acquired haemolytic anaemia— immune warm type
Blood

Idiopathic autoimmune haemolysis with antibody showing anti-ē specificity. A 5-year-old child with splenomegaly; haemoglobin 5.2 g/dl; MCV 94 fl; reticulocytes $610 \times 10^9/l$; and nucleated red cells $2.6 \times 10^9/l$. Gross anisocytosis, marked spherocytosis.

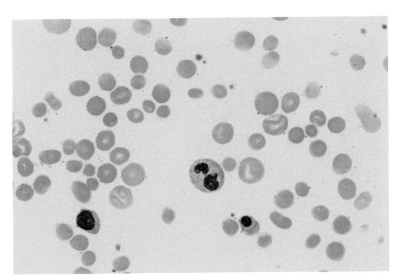

3.26 Acquired haemolytic anaemia— immune cold type
Blood

Gross agglutination at room temperature in a 7-year-old boy with mycoplasma pneumonia. There was associated haemolysis with a haemoglobin of 8 g/dl, and a marked reticulocytosis. Direct AHG test was positive with the red cells being coated with C4, C3b, and C3d. Serum contained a cold auto/panagglutinin with anti-I specificity.

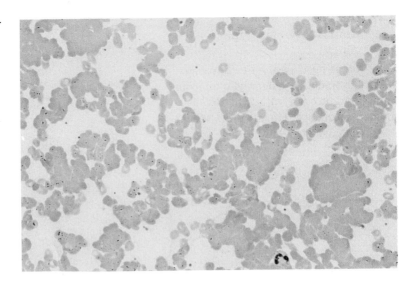

3.27 Acquired haemolytic anaemia— paroxysmal cold haemoglobinuria
Blood

PCH is occasionally seen in children following virus infections as an episode of acute haemolysis associated with the biphasic Donath–Landsteiner antibody with anti-P specificity. There are microagglutinates and there is often evidence of erythrophagocytosis by neutrophils.

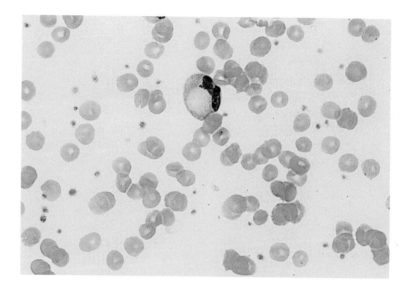

3.28 Secondary haemolytic anaemia—haemolytic uraemic syndrome
Blood

Marked red cell fragmentation associated with anaemia, thrombocytopenia, and renal failure but in the absence of disseminated intravascular coagulation. Girl of 5 years. The epidemic form is associated with endotoxins from enteric pathogenic Gram-negative bacteria.

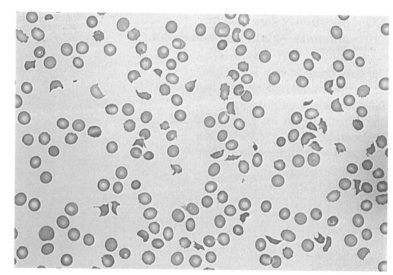

3.29 Secondary haemolytic anaemia—dapsone
Blood

Dapsone can put normal red cells under oxidative stress that they cannot withstand and a haemolytic anaemia results which shows the illustrated red cell poikilocytosis. Supravital staining would show the presence of Heinz bodies— clumps of denatured haemoglobin at the periphery of the cell.

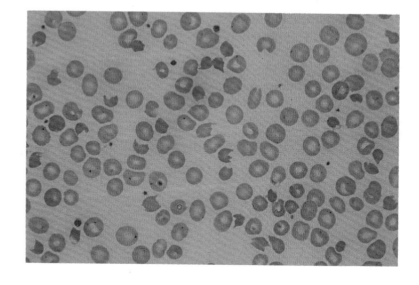

3.30 Secondary haemolytic anaemia mechanical haemolysis
Blood

Spherocytes, fragmented cells, and polychromasia. Platelet count and renal function normal. A 9-year-old with a Teflon graft to repair a ventricular septal defect.

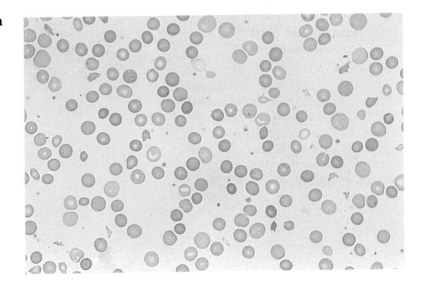

3.31 Secondary haemolytic anaemia—giant haemangioma
Blood

The Kasabach–Merritt syndrome, producing a microangiopathic haemolytic state due to the pathological microcirculation in the lesion. Red cell fragmentation and spherocytes are associated with thrombocytopenia.

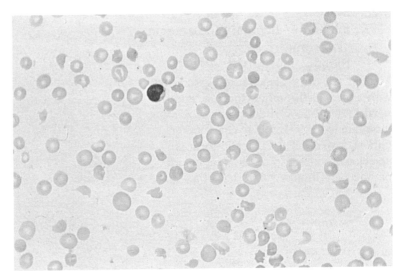

3.32 Secondary haemolytic anaemia—extensive burns
Blood

The film has a 'dirty' appearance due to cell debris and proteinaceous material. Partially burnt red cells have sphered, and others have completely lysed. Haemoglobin 6.2 g/dl. Six-month-old child in house fire.

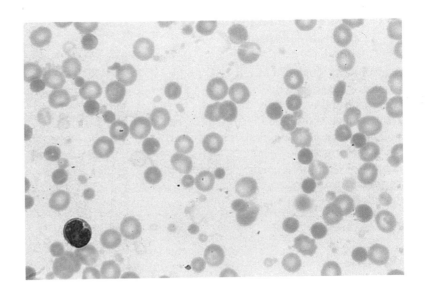

3.33   Haemolytic anaemia
Bone marrow

Normoblastic hyperplasia is the normal response to haemolysis from any cause. Its absence does not preclude haemolysis nor does its presence necessarily indicate it.

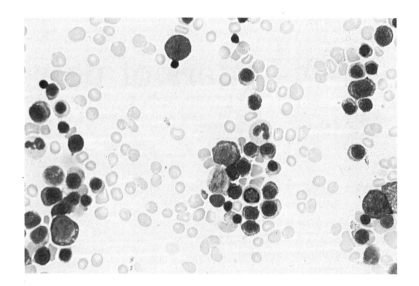

3.34   Post-splenectomy changes
Blood

Anisocytosis, poikilocytosis, target cells, thrombocytosis, and Howell–Jolly bodies. Twelve-year-old splenectomized for immune neutropenia.

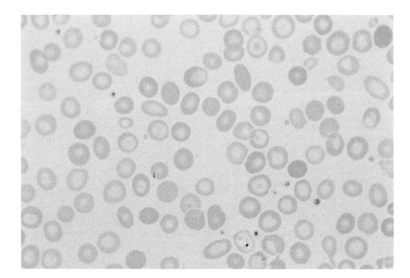

3.35   Congenital absence of spleen
Blood

Howell–Jolly bodies and irregularly contracted cells. An 18-month-old boy with an associated congenital heart defect—hypoplastic right outflow tract and partial situs inversus.

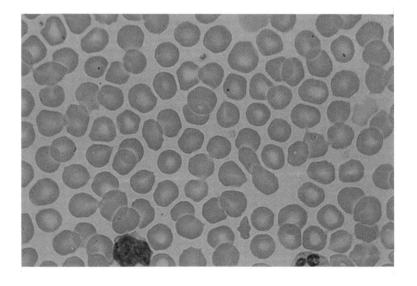

4
Disorders of polymorphonuclear leucocytes

4.1 Toxic granulation of neutrophils
Blood film

Dense neutrophil cytoplasmic granules are present and probably represent increased lysosomal content. There is a 'left shift' with reduced lobulation of the neutrophil nuclei. These features are present in patients with infections and other stresses (c.f. Chapter 14)

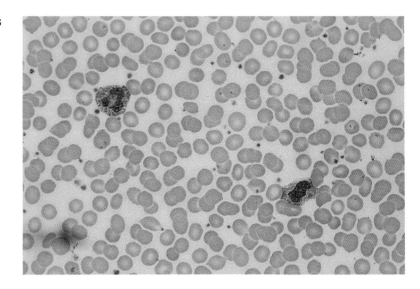

4.2 Toxic change due to septicaemia
Bone marrow

Toxic granulation is present in all the polymorph precursors and there is an increase in the more primitive forms such as myelocytes and promyelocytes giving a so-called 'left shift'.

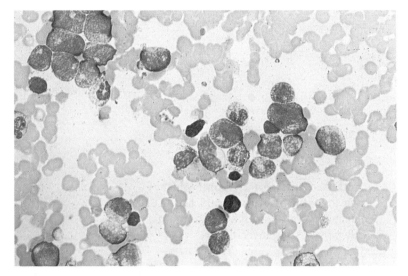

4.3 Pelger–Hüet anomaly
Blood film

This anomaly is transmitted in an autosomal fashion. Nuclei may be bilobed or oval shaped.

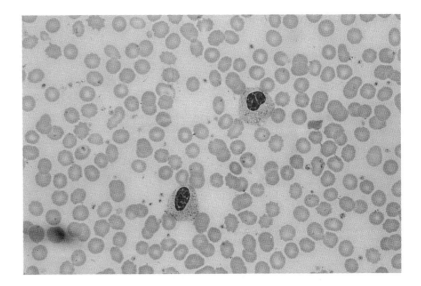

4.4 Pelger–Hüet anomaly
Blood film

The 'pince-nez' appearance of the neutrophils is shown in this plate. Neutrophils resembling these may also be seen in several acquired diseases such as myeloproliferative disorders and during sulphonamide therapy.

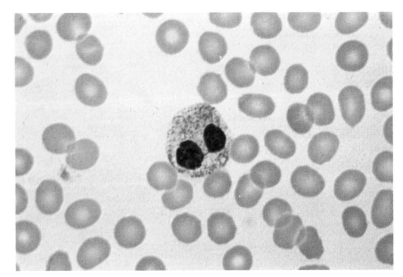

4.5 Neutrophil alkaline phosphatase (NAP)
Blood film

NAP activity is located in secondary and tertiary neutrophil granules and can be demonstrated by several techniques including the older azo-dye coupling and the newer BCIP–NBT method shown here. The intensity of the stain is an approximate measure of the cells' content of enzyme. Scoring on a 0–4 scale and counting 100 consecutive neutrophils the normal range in older patients is 35–100. In neonates scores tend to be higher (150–300). High scores also occur in infections, Down's syndrome, and leukaemoid reactions. Low scores are found in CGL in relapse, myeloblastic leukaemias, aplastic anaemia, and infectious mononucleosis.

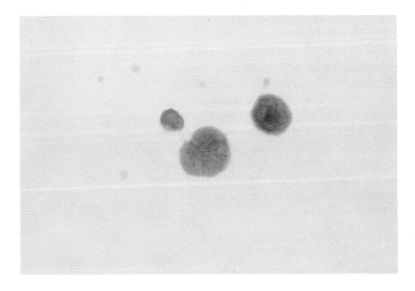

4.6 Specific granule deficiency.
Blood film

This is an extremely rare congenital disorder of neutrophil function. The patients present with recurrent bacterial infections and multiple abnormalities in neutrophil structure and composition. It is thought to be an autosomal recessive disorder. Protein deficiencies in azurophil granules (defensins) and light membranes suggest a common defect in the regulation of these proteins in myeloid cells. By light microscopy granules appear absent (by EM specific granule vesicles are absent or empty).

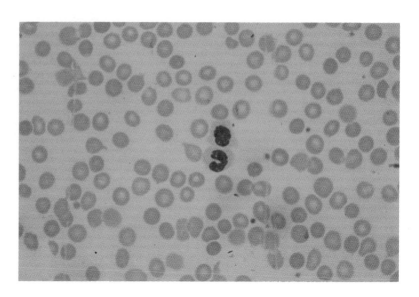

4.7 Eosinophilia due to toxoplasmosis
Blood film

Infection with *Toxoplasma gondii* is a cause of the 'infectious mononucleosis syndrome' in which generalized lymphadenopathy is associated with circulating atypical lymphocytes. In this case the more prominent feature was an eosinophilia.

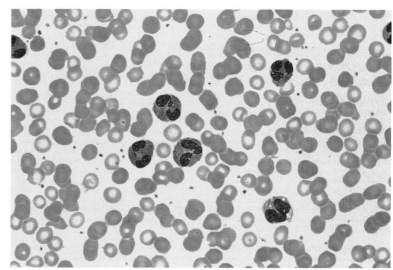

4.8 Chediak–Higashi syndrome
Blood film

Patients with this autosomal recessive disorder present with oculocutaneous albinism, fine light hair, and sometimes neurological problems and bleeding diathesis. The neutrophils (shown here), other white cells, as well as other tissue cells, show pyknotic nuclei and large irregular cytoplasmic granules. There may be profound pancytopenia and hepatosplenomegaly. Lymphoma-like disorders are also seen.

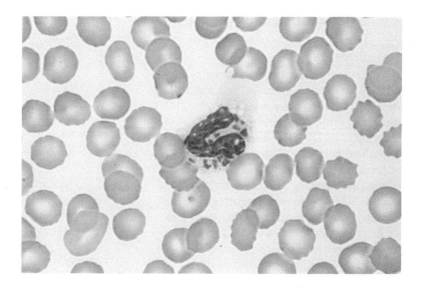

4.9 Chediak–Higashi syndrome
Blood, electron micrograph

Neutrophil containing abnormal granulation corresponding to the irregular granules shown in 4.8.

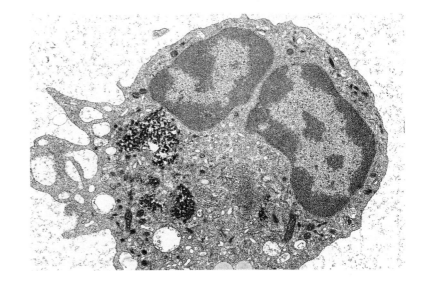

4.10 Chediak–Higashi syndrome
Bone marrow

The characteristic large (giant) eosinophilic granules are shown here together with the abnormal neutrophil granules. The giant eosinophilic granules are not so easily found in peripheral blood.

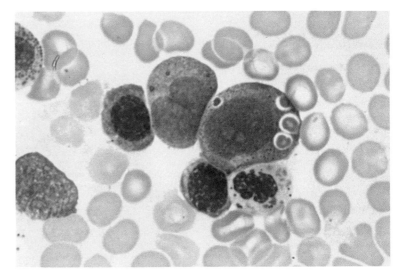

4.11 Nitro blue tetrazolium (NBT) test
Blood film

Neutrophils reduce the soluble tetrazolium salt to an insoluble blue–black formazan deposit. This reflects superoxide and singlet oxygen production by neutrophils during phagocytosis. The test can be used to detect both carriers and affected patients with chronic granulomatous disease. See Baehner and Nathan (1979). *New Eng. J. Med.*, **278**, 971 for details of method.

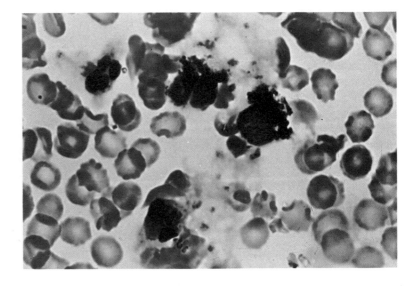

4.12   Opsonization experiment; positive result
Blood

Normal serum provokes complete ingestion of yeast granules by phagocytosis. This function is dependent upon two types of serum factor, IgA and C3, which coat the particles or bacteria.

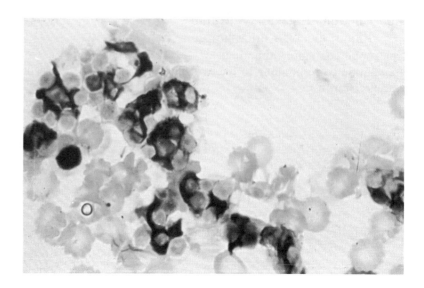

4.13   Opsonization experiment; negative result
Blood

Failure of yeast phagocytosis under these conditions occurs when there is a deficiency of C2, C3, C5, or a specific defect of humoral immunity. Recurrent and chronic pyogenic infections commonly result. Deficiency of mannose binding protein will also give a negative result, however, individuals with mannose binding protein deficiency may be asymptomatic.

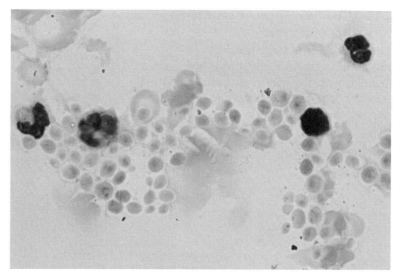

4.14   Systemic mastocytosis
Bone marrow

The sample is from a 3-year-old girl with moderate hepatosplenomegaly and developmental delay. She presented at age 13 months with fits sometimes associated with fever. She is said to have been 'flushed' at birth, perhaps as a result of histamine release from mast cells during the birth process.

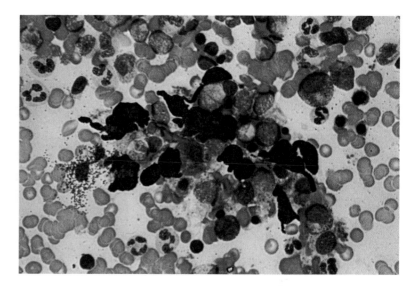

4.15   Systemic mastocytosis

Bone marrow; toluidine blue
The densely basophilic cytoplasm of the
mast cells makes recognition of the extent
of infiltration easier to appreciate.

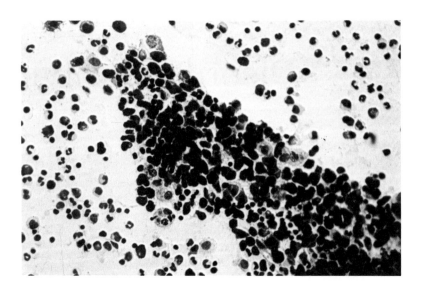

5
Disorders of lymphocytes

5.1 Pertussis (whooping cough)
Blood film

Typical haematological findings in pertussis include a very high lymphocytosis which may reach $100 \times 10^9/l$. In addition, the cells may have prominent nucleoli and basophilic cytoplasm as shown in this high-power view. The film appearance can be mistaken for lymphoblastic leukaemia.

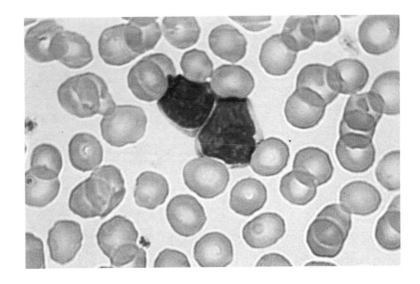

5.2 Infectious mononucleosis
Blood film

Infection with circulating EB virus causes a preponderance (more than 25 per cent) of circulating 'atypical mononuclear' cells which are mostly activated T-lymphocytes. Morphologically they have basophilic cytoplasm displaying characteristic darker 'crimped' areas where they impinge upon red cells. Nucleoli are often prominent and distinction of these cells from leukaemic blasts can sometimes be very difficult.

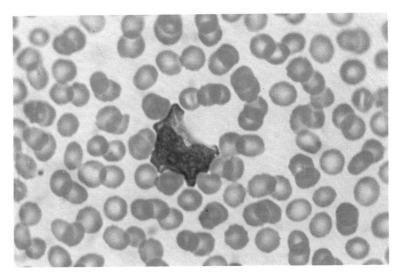

5.3 Infectious mononucleosis
Blood film

This plate shows another 'activated' lymphocyte with less prominent nucleoli than that shown in 5.2.

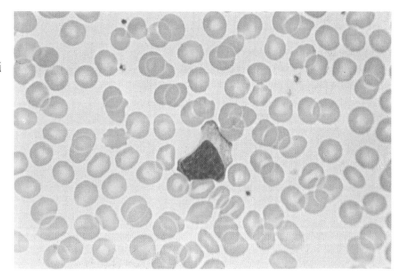

5.4 Persistent CMV infection
Blood film

Cytomegalovirus is another agent producing an infectious mononucleosis-like syndrome (compare 5.2 and 5.3). This plate shows a preponderance of mature lymphocytes with hypochromic red cells. This 2-year-old boy had a persistent infection and later developed abdominal lymphoma.

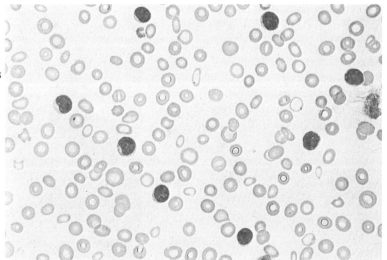

5.5 Persistent CMV infection
Blood film

The same patient's blood as shown in 5.4 again demonstrates a 'mature' lymphocytosis but some activated cells with basophilic cytoplasm are also seen.

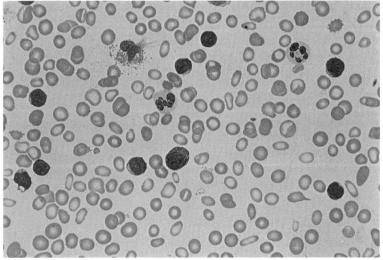

5.6   CMV infection
Blood film

These atypical lymphocytes show how CMV can be confused with infectious mononucleosis and even acute leukaemia, although the proportion of atypical forms is usually less than 25 per cent.

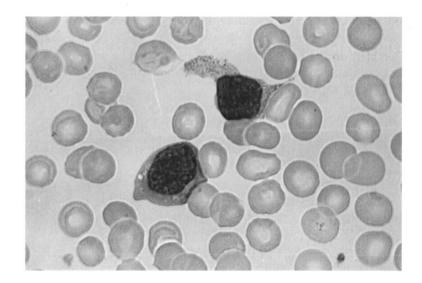

5.7   CMV infection in a 12-month-old infant
Bone marrow

The marrow shows 20 per cent lymphoblasts and 35 per cent lymphocytes and could easily be mistaken for leukaemia. CMV was cultured from the urine, throat, and blood buffy coat.

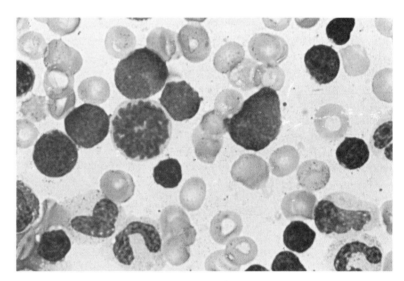

5.8   Castleman's syndrome
Bone marrow

A 7-year-old girl presented with PUO and normochromic–normocytic anaemia with red cell rouleaux. A retroperitoneal mass of lymph nodes was found on CT scan. Lymph node biopsy showed the plasma cell variant of this benign systemic lymphoproliferative disorder. Multiple organ involvement is common.

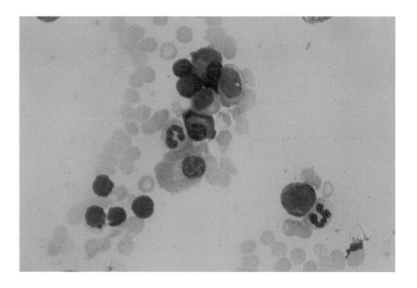

5.9 Castleman's syndrome
Marrow trephine biopsy; H&E
The marrow trephine histology demonstrates prominent plasma cells.

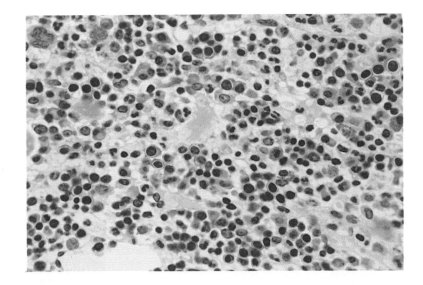

5.10 Castleman's syndrome
Lymph node; H&E
The lymph node histology also shows prominent plasma cells in this variant of the disorder.

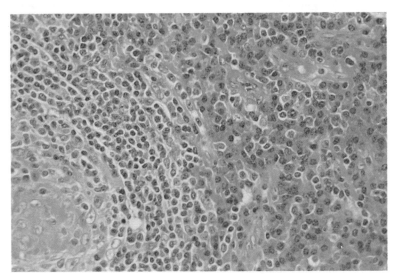

6
Platelet disorders

6.1 Idiopathic thrombocytopenic purpura (ITP)
Bone marrow

Large numbers of apparently immature and non-budding megakaryocytes are present. Although plentiful megakaryocytes are always seen in ITP, suggesting peripheral destruction of platelets, the morphological features are not diagnostic.

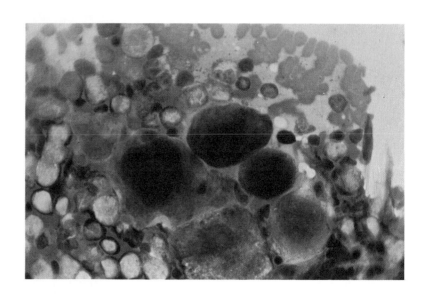

6.2 Bernard–Soulier syndrome
Blood film

This, along with the May–Hegglin anomaly and other rarer syndromes, e.g. that associated with nephritis and deafness, is one of the 'giant platelet' disorders. Inheritance is autosomal and incompletely recessive. As shown here, the platelets are almost as large as red cells. The long bleeding time in this condition results from the platelets' lack of a receptor site for Factor VIII associated protein (VIII^{Rag}).

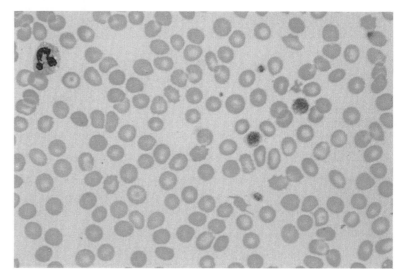

6.3 Bernard–Soulier syndrome
Blood film
Splenectomy was performed in this patient and a Howell–Jolly body is shown along with giant platelets. In fact, neither splenectomy nor corticosteroids are of clinical benefit.

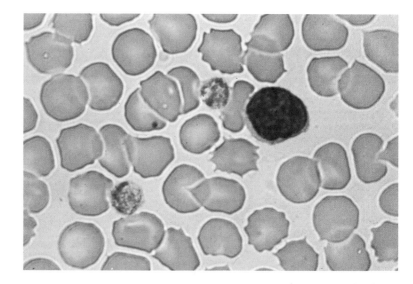

6.4 Bernard–Soulier syndrome
Blood film: electron micrograph
In this preparation the platelets can be seen to be almost equal in size to the white blood cells.

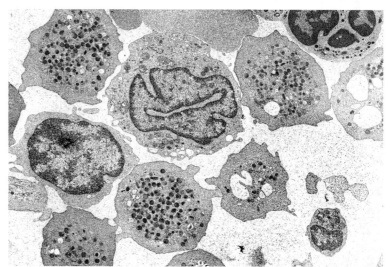

6.5 May–Hegglin anomaly
Blood film
Inheritance of this disorder is autosomal dominant and one-third of patients are thrombocytopenic. Neutrophil inclusions are present and resemble the Döhle bodies found in infected patients. The neutrophils show a 'sausage' shape of their nuclear lobes and giant platelets also occur.

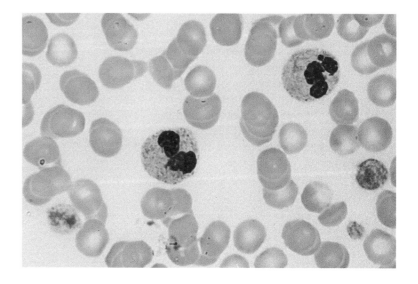

6.6 May–Hegglin anomaly
Blood film

Another example of the May–Hegglin anomaly.

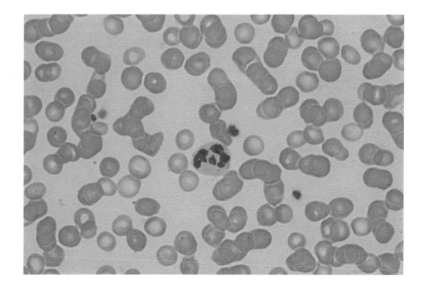

6.7 Wiskott–Aldrich syndrome
Blood film

Chronic thrombocytopenia, susceptibility to infection, and eczema characterize this sex-linked recessive disorder. The associated immunodeficiency is characterized by humoral and cellular abnormalities and susceptibility to lymphoreticular malignancies. This plate shows thrombocytopenia with typical very small platelets.

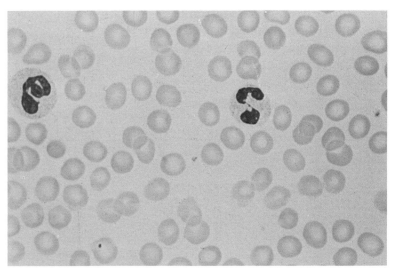

6.8 Thrombocytosis
Blood film

The platelet count in this blood sample was $1 \times 10^{12}/l$. There is marked anisothrombia. This patient had a reactive thrombocytosis following bleeding from a Meckel's diverticulum. Differential diagnosis is from: hyposplenism; infection; renal disease; myeloproliferative disorders; and other causes of marrow regeneration.

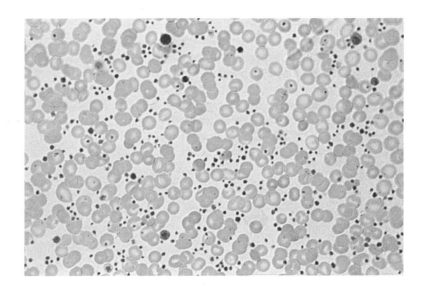

6.9 Grey platelet syndrome
Blood film

The patient presented with mild thrombocytopenia, mild bleeding problems and large agranular blue–grey platelets in the blood. Platelet aggregation is impaired but nucleotide and serotonin levels are normal. There is a profound abnormality in granule formation and a deficiency in α-granule substances, e.g. fibrinogen, β-thromboglobulin, platelet factor 4, coagulation factor V, and growth-promoting factor.

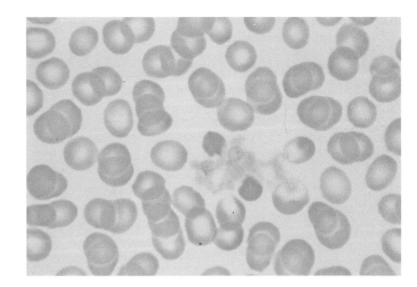

6.10 Electron micrograph of normal platelets
Blood

Normal platelets, seen here, contain dense bodies (few), which are not found in every platelet, α-granules, which are numerous and present in all platelets, as well as endoplasmic reticulum and mitochondria.

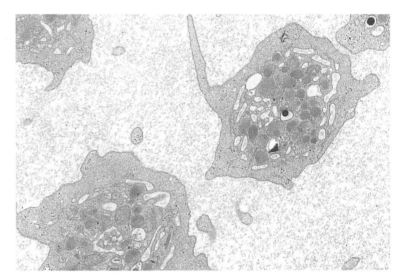

6.11 Electron micrograph of Grey platelets
Blood

The platelets in this disorder lack the α-granules of the normal, but otherwise the complement of organelles is normal. The lack of α-granules gives rise to the pale grey staining in routine blood films.

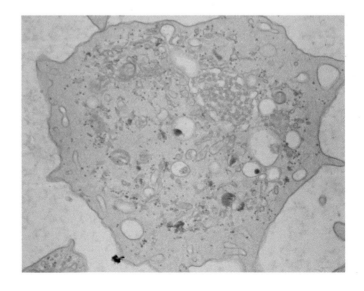

6.12   Giant platelets in liver disease on total parenteral nutrition (TPN)
Blood

This patient had cholestatic liver disease and was on TPN and had clotting abnormalities. Giant platelets were plentiful, and red cell targets were seen.

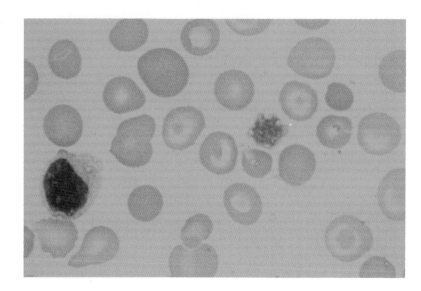

7
Acute lymphoblastic leukaemia (ALL)

The FAB classification of ALL

ALL is universally classified morphologically according to the criteria of a group of French, American, and British microscopists—the so-called FAB group.

FAB type L1 and type L2.

A zero or positive score = L1, a negative score = L2

Criteria*	Score†
High nuclear:cytoplasmic ratio ≥75 % of cells	+
Low nuclear:cytoplasmic ratio ≥25 % of cells	−
Nucleoli: 0 to 1 (small) ≥75 % of cells	+
Nucleoli: 1 or more (prominent) ≥25 % of cells	−
Irregular/convoluted nuclear membrane ≥25 % of cells	−
Large cells ≥50 % of cells ('large' = 2 × normal small lymphocyte)	−

  * The following are not scored: (1) intermediate or indeterminate criteria, (2) regular nuclear membrane in ≥75 per cent of cells, and (3) <50 per cent large cells, regardless of cell size heterogeneity.
  † Positive (+), or negative (−).

FAB type L3

L3 ALL is defined by its overall appearances, the key features being that the cells are large and have densely basophilic cytoplasm. Most have one or more prominent nucleoli. Prominent vacuolation is often present in most cells, usually to a greater extent than that seen in L1 and L2 disease.

Reference

Bennett, J.M., Catovsky, D., Daniel, M.T., Flandrin, G. (1981). The morphological classification of acute lymphoblastic leukaemia: concordance among observers and clinical correlations. *Br. J. Haematol.*, **47,** 553–561.

7.1   ALL FAB type L1
Bone marrow

The most frequent type of childhood leukaemia, the blasts are small and lymphocytoid. There is a high nuclear:cytoplasmic ratio and nucleoli are generally not visible. L1 morphology is seen in all immunologically defined ALL subtypes except B-ALL; most commonly it is associated with CD10 positivity, with or without cytoplasmic immunoglobulin. Hyperdiploidy (>50 chromosomes) is also more common in L1 disease.

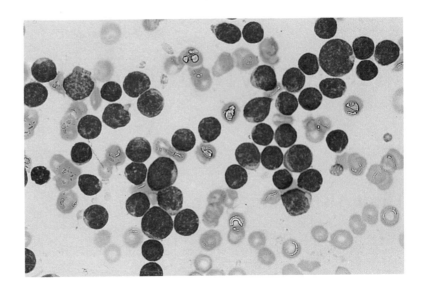

7.2   ALL FAB type L1
Bone marrow

Another example to show variable morphology.

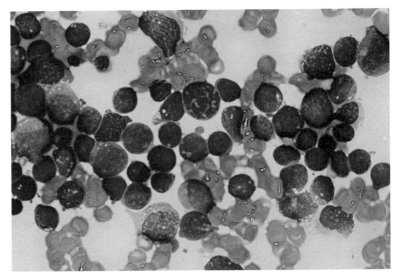

7.3   ALL FAB type L1
Bone marrow

Another example to show variable size.

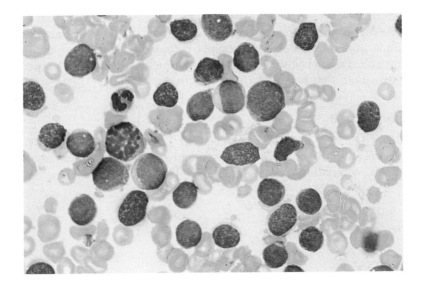

7.4 ALL FAB type L1 with vacuoles
Bone marrow

Vacuoles are found in the blasts from around 25 per cent of cases of childhood ALL other than those with L3 disease. They are thus not confined to the L3 subtype. They are associated with periodic acid–Schiff positivity, CD10 positivity, and a low circulating white cell count. Patients in this group have a prognostic advantage with current therapeutic schedules. Vacuoles are occasionally seen in L2 disease.

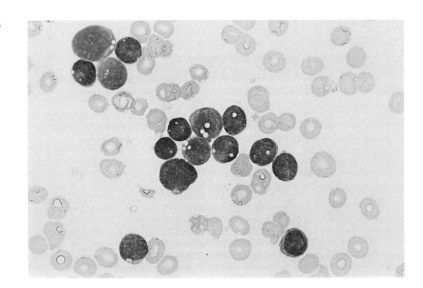

7.5 ALL FAB type L1 with 'hand mirror' cells
Bone marrow

The curious but striking amoeboid configuration of blast cells in some leukaemias has been likened to a hand mirror. The significance, if any, of this is unclear. Conflicting claims for prognostic significance has been made, though more have suggested it to be an adverse feature. The frequency of cases with > 10 per cent hand mirrors is low, below 5 per cent. They are not confined to L1 ALL.

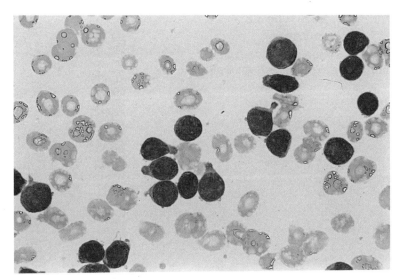

7.6 ALL FAB type L1 with granules
Bone marrow

Up to 7 per cent of cases of ALL will show peroxidase and Sudan black-negative azurophilic granules in some cells, the nature and importance of which are presently unknown. They are occasionally sufficiently striking to cause confusion with acute myeloblastic leukaemia (see Chapter 8).

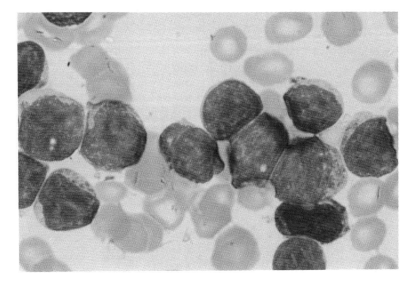

7.7   ALL FAB type L2
   Bone marrow

L2 ALL accounts for 10–15 per cent of all cases and is defined by the presence of a low nuclear:cytoplasmic ratio, conspicuous nucleoli, irregular nuclear outline, and bigger blast cells (see above). It is associated with periodic acid–Schiff negativity, and arises more often in older children. L2 disease may be more resistant to treatment and has a higher remission–induction failure rate.

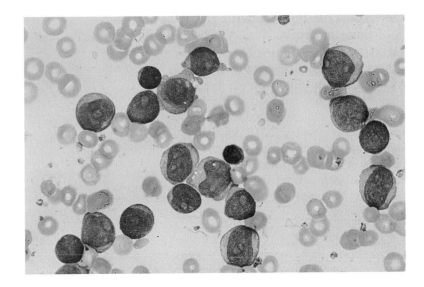

7.8   ALL FAB type L2
   Bone marrow

Another example to show variable morphology (prominent nucleoli).

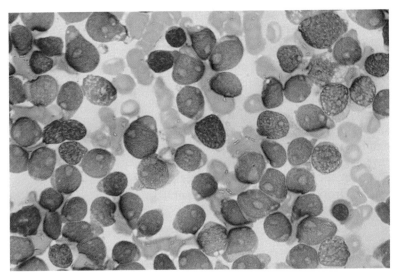

7.9   ALL FAB type L2
   Bone marrow

An example with large cells showing nucleoli, a low nuclear:cytoplasmic ratio, and some nuclear convolution.

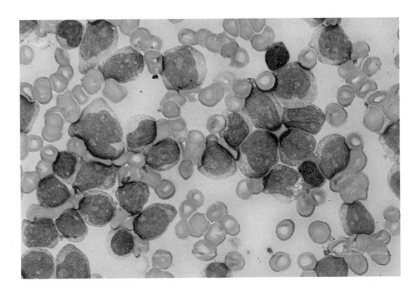

7.10 ALL T-cell type, peripheral blood
Blood

The T-cell subtype of ALL can often give rise to very high white cell counts. The count in this example was $450 \times 10^9/l$. The appearance of the cells in the blood can be different from that in the marrow. FAB typing should always and only be carried out on bone marrow. The cells illustrated are large and some show nuclear convolution.

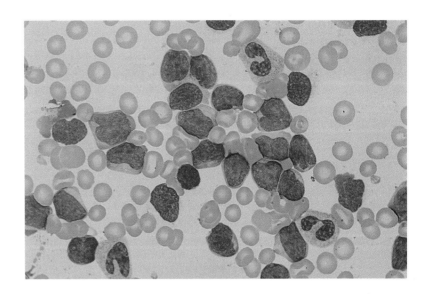

7.11 ALL T-cell type, bone marrow
Bone marrow

Marrow from the patient illustrated in 7.10. The cells appear smaller and more dense than in the peripheral blood, and would classify as FAB type L1.

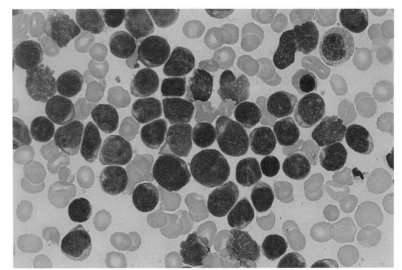

7.12 ALL FAB type L3
Bone marrow

The rarest type of ALL, L3 accounts for <1 per cent of cases. It is nearly always of B-cell immunophenotype, a type which does not arise in L1 or L2 disease. The cells are large, densely basophilic, heavily vacuolated, and variably have conspicuous nucleoli. It is associated with a non-random chromosome abnormality (t(8;14)). The vacuoles are usually positive for Oil Red O.

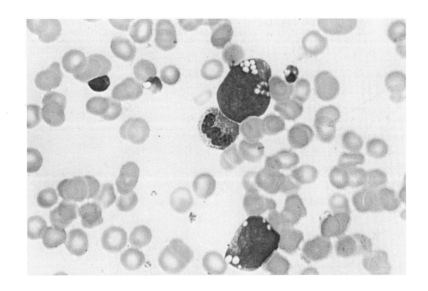

7.13   ALL FAB type L3
Bone marrow
A further example.

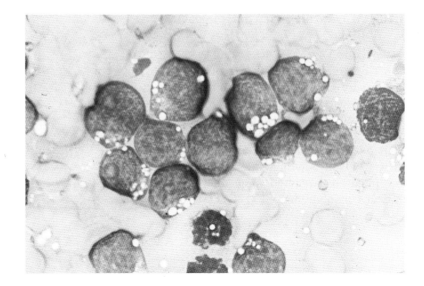

7.14   ALL FAB type L3
Bone marrow
A further example where the characteristic morphology is less striking. Distinction from other types of ALL is not always easy.

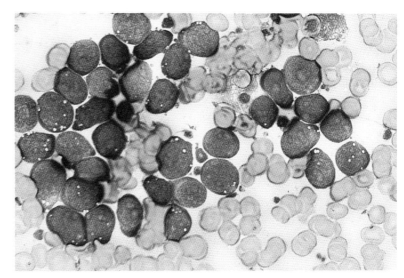

7.15   ALL cytochemistry
Bone marrow; PAS reaction
periodic acid–Schiff (PAS) positivity in 'blocks' and coarse granules is commonly found in childhood ALL—between 50 and 60 per cent of cases. Vacuoles (other than in L3 disease) are associated with PAS positivity, as is CD10 reactivity, a low white count, and L1 morphology. L2 disease is more often negative. Strong PAS positivity thus associates with good prognostic features.

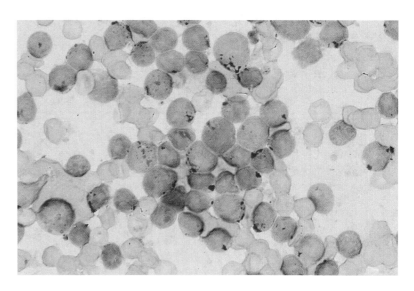

7.16 ALL cytochemistry
   Bone marrow; acid phosphatase
Non-diffuse acid phosphatase positivity is
found typically in T-cell ALL as in this
case. It is not exclusively so, being
negative in 5–10 per cent of T-cell cases
and positive in a third of non-T diseases.
Positivity in non-T ALL is usually much
weaker than in T-ALL, but not
invariably.

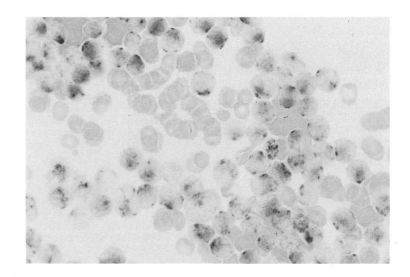

7.17 ALL cytochemistry
   Bone marrow; Oil Red O
Lymphoblasts, particularly the heavily
vacuolated L3 type (though not
exclusively so), take up the lipid stain Oil
Red O. The stain is seldom helpful in
distinguishing subtypes of ALL, or in
distinguishing ALL from other
leukaemias.

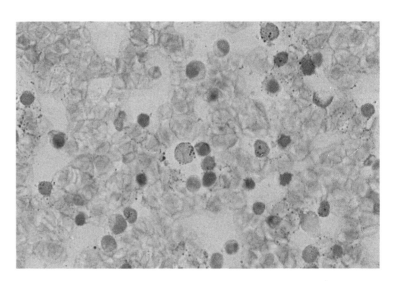

7.18 ALL marrow histology
   Trephine biopsy; HE stain
Diffuse total marrow replacement with
loss of fat spaces is the commonest finding
in childhood ALL.

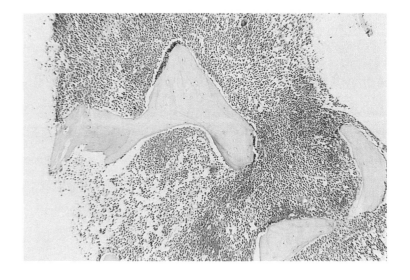

7.19   ALL marrow histology
Trephine biopsy; reticulin stain
Around 10–20 per cent of cases have sufficient secondary marrow fibrosis to make aspiration very difficult.

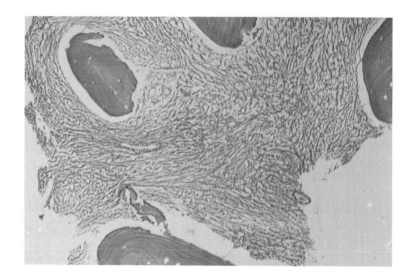

7.20   ALL marrow histology
Trephine biopsy; HE stain
Patchy infiltration with preservation of normal architecture is sometimes seen in the so-called 'lymphoma-leukaemia' syndrome, typical of T-cell ALL as in this case.

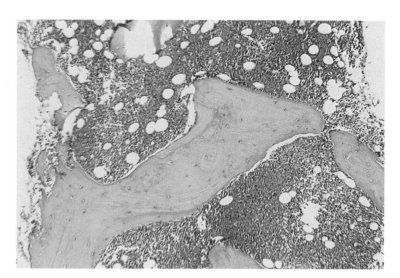

7.21   Extramedullary ALL—CNS
Cytocentrifuge preparation; cerebrospinal fluid
CNS leukaemia as an isolated relapse; cell count $100/mm^3$ ($0.1 \times 10^9/l$). The morphology may be distorted in such preparations and appear different from that seen in blood or marrow smears. Where very few white cells are present (< 5–$10/mm^3$), it can be very difficult to be certain of their nature on cytospin preparations. In such circumstances it may be impossible to make a diagnosis. The presence of mitotic figures is usually sinister.

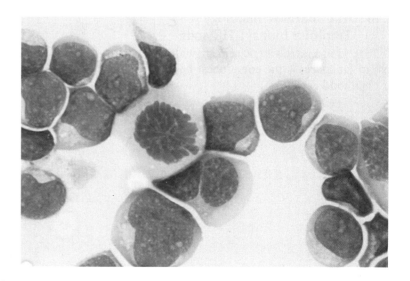

7.22 Extramedullary ALL—CNS
Cytocentrifuge preparation;
cerebrospinal fluid

CNS leukaemia as part of a multi-site
relapse. Cell count $2000/mm^3$ $(2 \times 10^9/l)$.
With this degree of infiltration there is no
diagnostic difficulty.

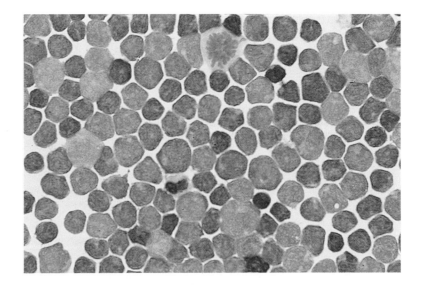

7.23 Extramedullary ALL—CNS
Paraffin section of superficial
cerebral cortex post mortem;
H&E stain

Dense meningeal infiltration extending
down the intracerebral perivascular
meningeal sheaths but no direct invasion
of brain tissue. Even in advanced disease
direct neural invasion is unusual

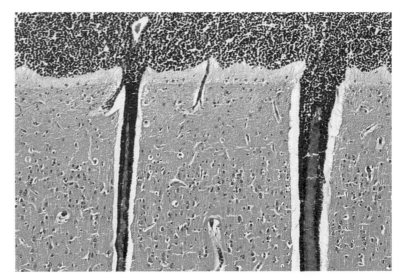

**7.24 Extramedullary ALL—pleural
effusion**
Cytocentrifuge preparation;
pleural fluid

A malignant pleural effusion in T-ALL.
Such effusions are more frequent in the
'leukaemia–lymphoma' syndrome typical
of T-ALL and (to a lesser extent) B-ALL.

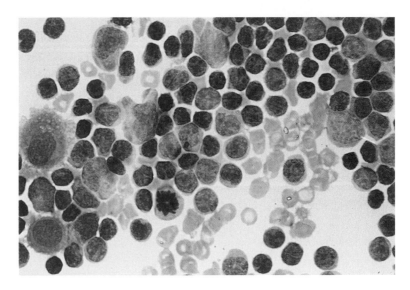

7.25   Extramedullary ALL—anterior chamber of eye
Microneedle aspirate of anterior chamber

On rare occasions this complication, presenting as a hypopyon, can be an isolated phenomenon without evidence of disease elsewhere. It can be the sole site of detectable active disease.

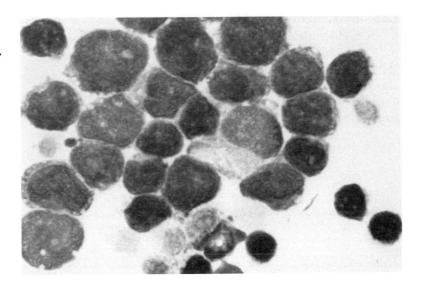

7.26   Extramedullary ALL—testicular infiltration, paraffin section; H&E stain

A common site of isolated late relapse. The section shows a light interstitial infiltrate between the seminiferous tubules in an elective biopsy done at the end of treatment in a boy thought to be in complete remission.

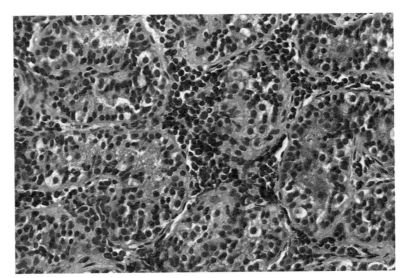

7.27   Extramedullary ALL—testicular infiltration
Touch preparation from testicular biopsy

Dabbing a fresh biopsy specimen on a slide and using a Romanowsky stain can demonstrate the presence of lymphoblasts.

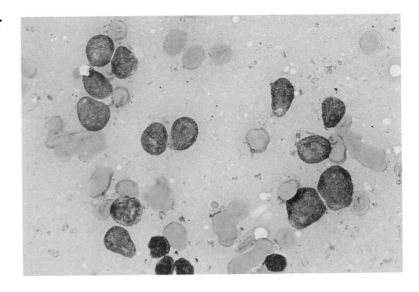

7.28   Extramedullary ALL—testicular infiltration
Touch preparation from testicular biopsy
A further example.

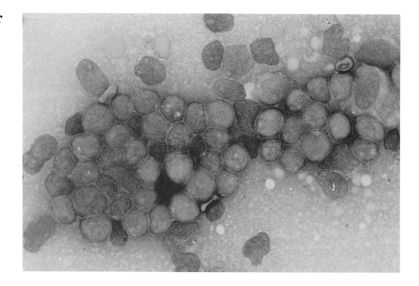

7.29   Biphenotypic relapse of ALL
Bone marrow
Rarely relapse of ALL may show features of both ALL and AML. There can be two populations evident morphologically as in this case.

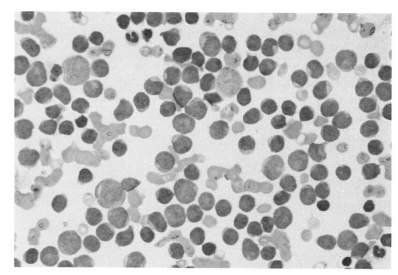

7.30   Interphase cytogenetic studies
Bone marrow
Fluorescence *in situ* hybridization techniques can show cytogenetic abnormalities in non-dividing cells even on old stored marrow slides. The example illustrated shows trisomy for the X chromosome in the malignant cells of a girl at the time of presentation of ALL. The slide was over 3 years old at the time of study, though had been kept unfixed and frozen at −20 °C.

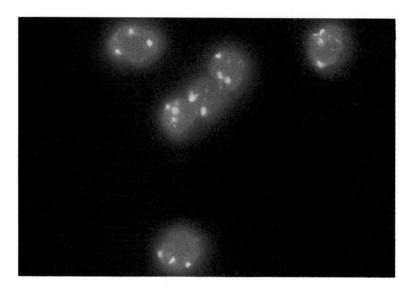

7.31 ALL; 'rebound' lymphocytosis
Bone marrow (low power)
Extreme degrees of lymphocytosis with an excess of blasts are very common in patients who have recently stopped chemotherapy. It cannot be emphasized strongly enough that mistakes in marrow interpretation are frequently made at this stage and extreme caution must always be exercised.

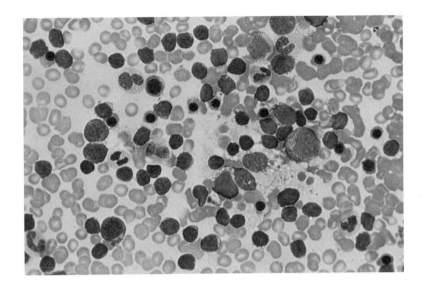

7.32 ALL; 'rebound' lymphocytosis
Bone marrow (high power)
A high-power view of the patient's marrow shown in 7.31 shows the presence of a lymphoblast and a number of lymphocytes. This phenomenon can persist for over a year and has no demonstrable prognostic significance. These 'normal' blasts are terminal deoxynucleotidyl transferase (TdT) positive and express the CD10 antigen.

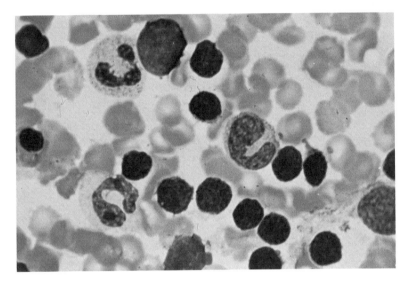

8
Acute non-lymphoblastic leukaemia (ANNL, or acute myeloid leukaemia, AML)

The FAB classification of ANLL (AML)

ANLL is universally classified morphologically according to the criteria of a group of French, American, and British microscopists—the so-called FAB group. The system can be summarized as follows:

FAB type M0

1. Obvious acute leukaemia where blast cells are devoid of granules. Less than 3 per cent peroxidase or Sudan black-positive. Negative for lymphocyte-related clusters of differentiation; positive for at least one myeloid antigen.

FAB type M1

1. Blast cells, agranular and granular types (types I and II) more than 90 per cent of non-erythroid cells. At least 3 per cent of these peroxidase or Sudan black-positive.
2. Remaining 10 per cent of cells (or less) are maturing granulocytes or monocytes.

FAB type M2

1. Sum of agranular and granular blasts (types I and II) is from 30–89 per cent of non-erythroid cells.
2. Monocytic cells, less than 20 per cent.
3. Granulocytes from promyelocytes to mature polymorphs, more than 10 per cent.

FAB type M3

1. Majority of cells are abnormal promyelocytes with heavy granulation.
2. Characteristic cells containing bundles of Auer rods ('faggots') invariably present.
3. A hypogranular variant occurs where the cells show similar morphology without heavy azurophil granulation. Occasional 'faggot' cells can usually be found.

FAB type M4

1. In the marrow, blasts more than 30 per cent of non-erythroid cells.
2. Sum of myeloblasts, promyelocytes, myelocytes and later granulocytes is between 30 and 80 per cent of non-erythroid cells.
3. More than 20 per cent of non-erythroid cells are monocyte lineage.
4. If monocytic cells exceed 80 per cent, diagnosis is M5.

Note:
(a) If marrow findings as above and peripheral blood monocytes (all types) are more than $5.0 \times 10^9/l$, the diagnosis is M4.
(b) If monocyte count less than $5.0 \times 10^9/l$, M4 can be confirmed on basis of serum lysozyme or esterase staining.
(c) The diagnosis of M4 is confirmed if more than 20 per cent of marrow precursors are monocytes (confirmed by special stains).

FAB type M4 with eosinophilia

1. Eosinophils more than 5 per cent of non-erythroid cells in marrow.
2. Eosinophils are abnormal.
3. Eosinophils are chloroacetate-esterase and PAS-positive.

FAB type M5

1. Eighty per cent or more of marrow non-erythroid cells are monoblasts, promono-cytes or monocytes.
2. M5a, 80 per cent of monocytic cells are monoblasts.
3. M5b, less than 80 per cent of monocytic cells are monoblasts, remainder are pre-dominantly promonocytes and monocytes.

FAB type M6

1. The erythroid component of the marrow exceeds 50 per cent of all nucleated cells.
2. Thirty per cent or more of the remaining non-erythroid cells are agranular or granular blasts (types I and II).

Note: if more than 50 per cent erythroid cells but less than 30 per cent blasts, diagnosis becomes myelodysplastic syndrome.

FAB type M7

1. Thirty per cent at least of nucleated cells are blasts.
2. Blasts identified by platelet peroxidase on EM, or by monoclonal antibodies to platelet antigens such as CD 42 or CD 61.
3. Increased reticulin is common.

References

1. Bennett, J.A., Catovsky, D., Daniel, M.T., Flandrin, G., Galton, D.A.G., Gralnick, H.R., Sultan, and C. (1985). Proposed revised criteria for the classification of acute myeloid leukemia. *Ann. Intern. Med.*, **103**, 626–9.
2. Bennett, J.A., Catovsky, D., Daniel, M.T., Flandrin, G., Galton, D.A.G., Gralnick, H.R., and Sultan, C. (1991). Proposal for the recognition of minimally differentiated acute myeloid leukaemia (AML M0). *Br. J. Haematol.*, **78**, 325–9.

8.1 Acute myeloid leukaemia FAB type M0
Bone marrow

Nearly all agranular undifferentiated blasts. Differentiation from ALL type L2 on Romanowsky-stained morphology can be difficult or impossible. The latter is more common in children. Immunological typing is needed to make a definitive diagnosis. Should be negative for lymphoid clusters of differentiation and positive for at least one myeloid antigen (CD 13 or 33).

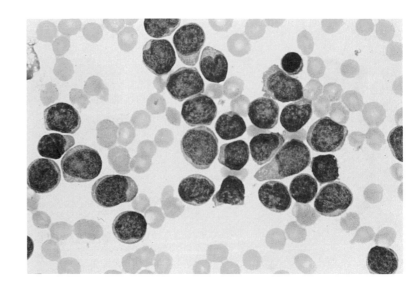

8.2 Acute myeloid leukaemia FAB type M1
Bone marrow

Myeloid differentiation is more clear than in M0, with granules and occasional Auer rods (altered primary granules) being visible.

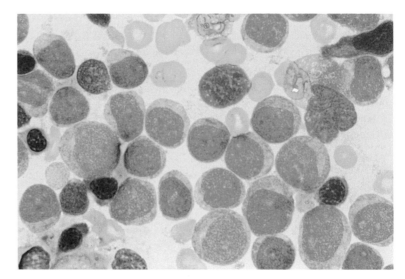

8.3 Acute myeloid leukaemia FAB type M1
Bone marrow

Close-up of a Romanowsky-stained cell containing an Auer rod.

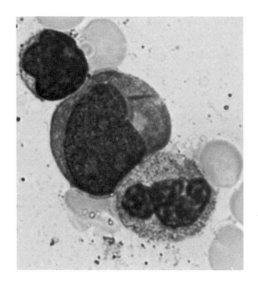

8.4   Acute myeloid leukaemia FAB type M1
Bone marrow; myeloperoxidase stain

Usually weak but unequivocal positivity is seen in over 3 per cent of cells, and the stain picks out Auer rods that may not be so easily visible on Romanowsky staining.

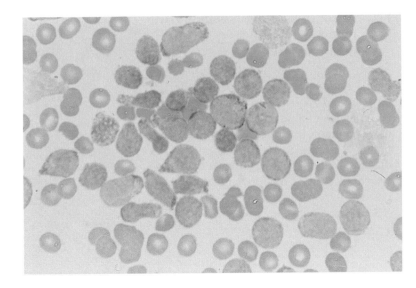

8.5   Acute myeloid leukaemia FAB type M2
Bone marrow

Differentiated from type M1 by having more blasts showing obvious granulation. Auer rods may or may not be present. Patients with the (8;21) chromosome translocation show M2 morphology.

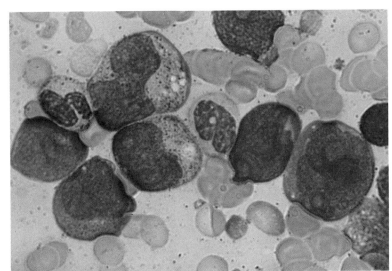

8.6   Acute myeloid leukaemia FAB type M2
Bone marrow; peroxidase stain

A greater proportion of cells staining with greater intensity than in type M1 (8.4). Auer rods appear thicker showing intense peroxidase activity.

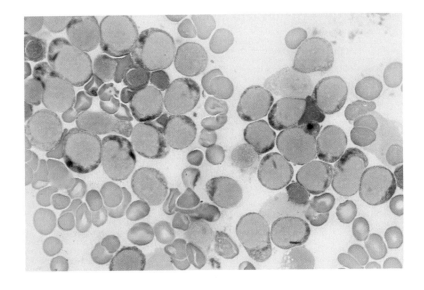

8.7 Acute myeloid leukaemia FAB type M2

Bone marrow; Sudan black stain
Peroxidase and Sudan black stains closely correlate with each other. The staining intensity may differ. Sudan black may be a preferable technique, as peroxidase staining requires the use of potential carcinogens to get the best results.

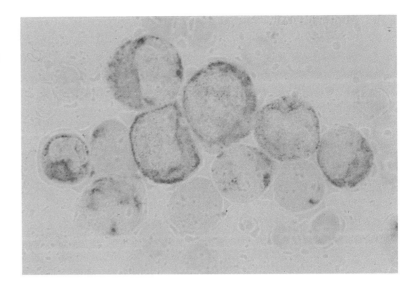

8.8 Acute myeloid leukaemia FAB type M2

Bone marrow; Sudan black stain
Sudan black, like peroxidase, can show up Auer rods and make them more easily visible than on Romanowsky staining.

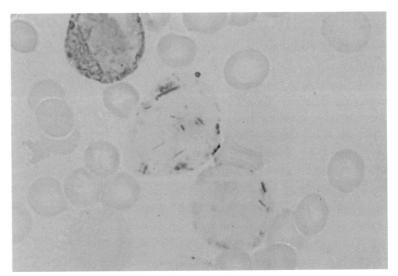

8.9 Acute myeloid leukaemia FAB type M3

Bone marrow
Promyelocytic leukaemia. Dense azurophil granules fill the cytoplasm, with many Auer rods. The nucleus shows variable shape and size within the cell. Such cells are strongly peroxidase-positive and sudanophilic. Characteristically there is a t(15;17) karyotype.

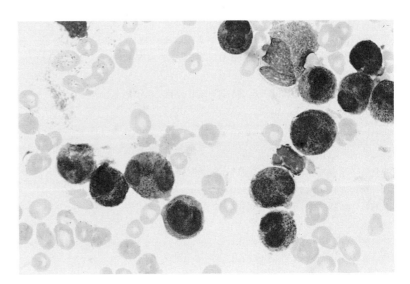

8.10 Acute myeloid leukaemia FAB type M3
Blood film

A high-power view of a malignant promyelocyte showing numerous Auer rods—the so-called 'faggot' cell.

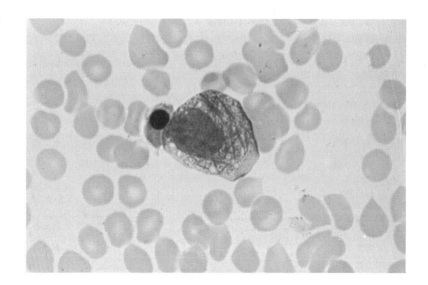

8.11 Acute myeloid leukaemia FAB type M3 variant
Blood film

A hypogranular variant of M3 is recognized which, like the typical variety, can cause a consumption coagulopathy, but where the cells are not so strikingly granular. It also shows the t(15;17) karyotype. The cells show nuclear convolution and are mostly not heavily granulated, but there are a few 'faggot' cells to be found.

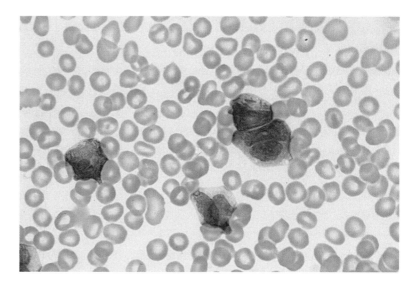

8.12 Acute myelomonocytic leukaemia (AMML)—FAB type M4
Blood film

M4 AMML is defined by 20–80 per cent non-erythroid cells in the marrow being monocyte-related and (typically) the circulating monoblast/monocyte count being $> 5 \times 10^9/l$. A characteristic clinical feature of monocyte related leukaemias in children with permanent teeth is gingival hypertrophy.

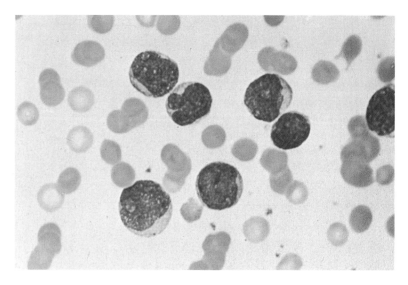

8.13 Acute myelomonocytic leukaemia—FAB type M4
Bone marrow

Blasts are > 30 per cent of non-erythroid cells, and > 20 per cent but < 80 per cent show monocytic features (cytochemically and/or immunologically).

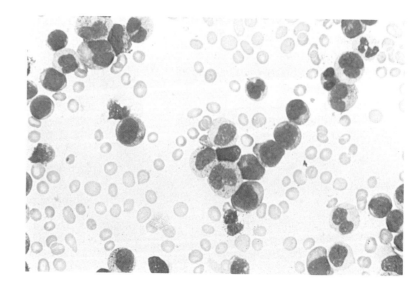

8.14 Acute myelomonocytic leukaemia—FAB type M4
Bone marrow; combined esterase stain

Combined chloroacetate and α-naphthyl acetate esterase stain with fast blue BB for coupling the former and hexazonium pararosanilin for the latter. The monocytic (brown) component is admixed with the granulocyte (blue) component.

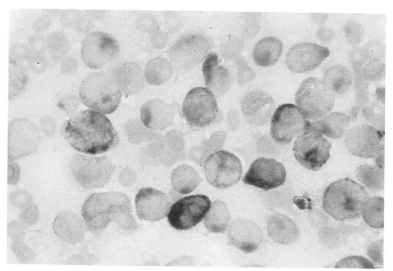

8.15 Acute myelomonocytic leukaemia with eosinophils (FAB type M4EO)
Bone marrow

The presence of numerous atypical eosinophils marks this variant of M4 AMML which is also associated with a specific chromosome abnormality (inv/del (16)(q22)).

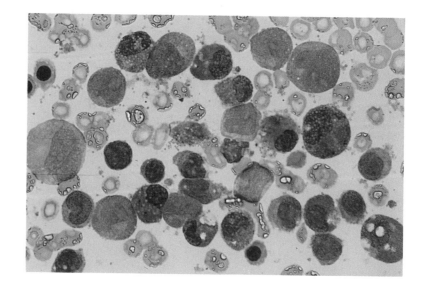

8.16   Acute monocytic leukaemia (AMoL)—FAB type M5
Bone marrow

Over 80 per cent of blasts show monocytic lineage, cytochemically and immunologically. Romanowsky morphology is hard to distinguish in some cases from M1 or L2.

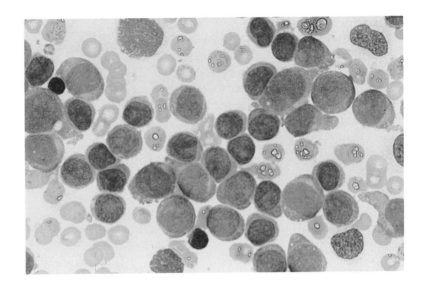

8.17   Acute monocytic leukaemia
Bone marrow; combined esterase stain

The same case as 8.16 stained as in 8.14. There are no chloroacetate esterase-positive cells present—only those with α-naphthyl acetate esterase.

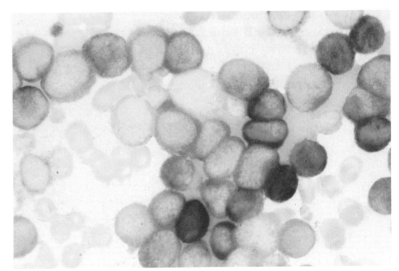

8.18   Acute monocytic leukaemia with erythrophagocytosis
Bone marrow

A variant of M5 AMoL that is characterized by erythrophagocytosis and a specific chromosome abnormality (t(8;16)(p11;p13)).

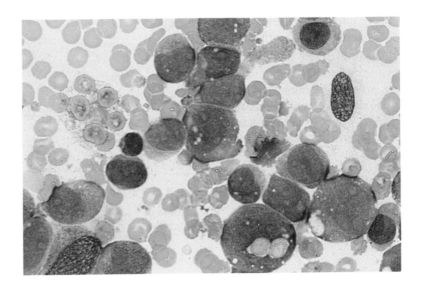

8.19 Acute erythroleukaemia (AEL)—FAB type M6
Bone marrow
Criteria for this diagnosis include: > 30 per cent of non-erythroid cells are type 1 or 2 blast cells (see 8.1 and 8.5); > 50 per cent of all cells are erythroid. This category of disease is very rare in childhood. The photograph is of the disease in a 15-year-old.

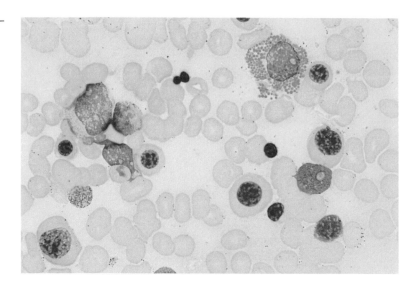

8.20 Acute erythroleukaemia
Blood film; PAS reaction
Erythroblasts in M6 AEL show coarse or diffuse variable to strong periodic acid–Schiff (PAS) positivity in around 50 per cent of cases.

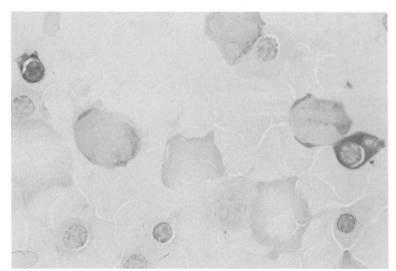

8.21 Acute megakaryoblastic leukaemia (AMKL)—FAB type M7
Bone marrow
AMKL cannot be diagnosed on morphology alone, and requires the demonstration of platelet peroxidase on electron microscopy or antigens recognized by platelet or factor VIII-specific mono- or polyclonal antibodies. Cytochemical patterns vary; there may be non-diffuse α-naphthyl acetate esterase and/or acid phosphatase. Blasts vary in size and may have cytoplasmic blebs as in the case illustrated. The disease is rare in normal children, but is seen more frequently in those with Down's syndrome.
Chromosome 21 may be abnormal in M7 blasts from non-Down's children.

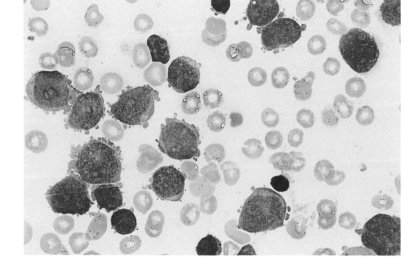

8.22 Acute megakaryoblastic leukaemia—marrow fibrosis
Trephine biopsy; reticulin stain
Associated secondary marrow fibrosis is a common feature of M7 AMKL and may make aspiration extremely difficult.

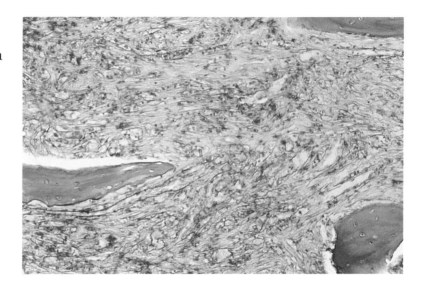

8.23 Acute megakaryoblastic leukaemia—platelet glycoprotein expression
Bone marrow
Alkaline phosphatase anti-alkaline phosphatase (APAAP) technique showing strong positivity for CD42 (Gplb) in a blast cell from a patient with M7 AMKL.

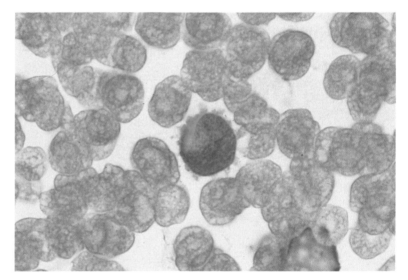

8.24 Acute megakaryoblastic leukaemia—factor VIII antigen expression
Trephine biopsy
Immunoperoxidase staining of factor VIII antigen in blasts in a section of marrow from a child with M7 AMKL.

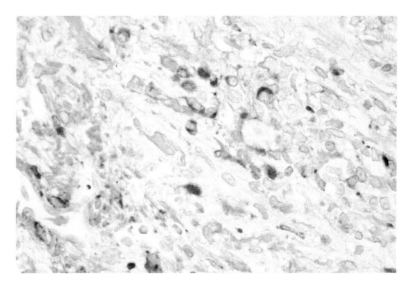

8.25 Acute myeloid leukaemia—CNS relapse
CSF cytocentrifuge

CNS relapse does rarely occur in AML and can be diagnosed on a cytocentrifuge preparation from CSF as with ALL. Numerous myeloblasts and some monocytes are seen.

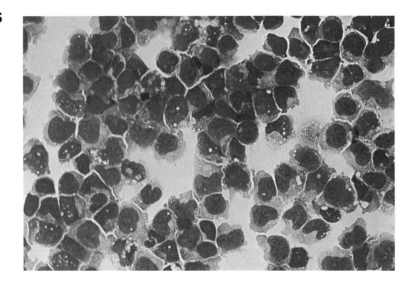

8.26 Acute myeloid leukaemia—CNS relapse
CSF cytocentrifuge

A further example from an infant with congenital leukaemia (type M5). See Chapter 14.

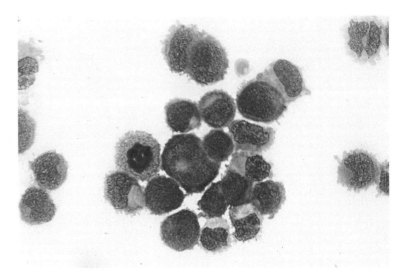

8.27 Chronic granulocytic leukaemia—myeloid blast crisis
Blood film

The chronic phase of CGL often terminates as 'blast crisis'—either lymphoid, myeloid, or mixed. This particular girl presented with a myeloid blast crisis 5 years from diagnosis. Many myeloblasts are present along with other abnormal myeloid precursors including degranulated basophils and eosinophils.

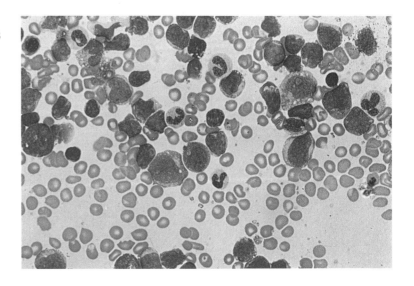

8.28 Chronic granulocytic leukaemia—lymphoid blast crisis
Bone marrow

Blast cells from a 4-year-old boy with Ph[1]-positive CGL that transformed after 18 months into acute leukaemia showing additional chromosome abnormalities together with the immunophenotype of 'common' ALL (CD10 positive). He returned to the chronic phase after standard ALL therapy.

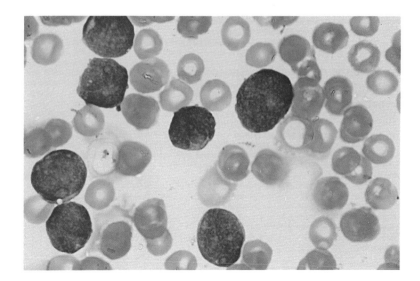

9
Myeloproliferative disorders

9.1 Refractory anaemia
Blood film

The patient had a transfusion dependent reticulocytopenic anaemia. There were no blasts in the blood but the red cells showed marked anisocytosis with occasional target forms and polychromatic macrocytes. The white cells and platelets were normal.

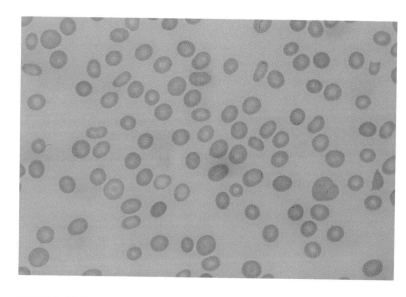

9.2 Refractory anaemia
Bone marrow

This type of myelodysplasia may not progress to leukaemia or RAEB(t). Diagnosis depends on the lack of other features of myelodysplasia and is essentially one of exclusion (e.g. rule out congenital dyserythropoietic anaemia). The marrow in this case showed marked dyserythropoiesis. A clonal cytogenetic abnormality usually clinches the diagnosis.

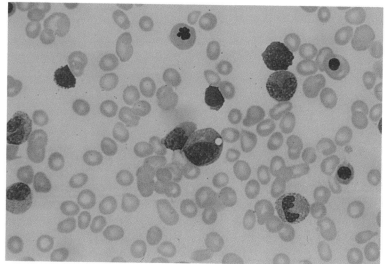

9.3 RAEB with monosomy 7
Blood film

A childhood syndrome characterized by hepatosplenomegaly, recurrent infections, myeloproliferation and refractory anaemia with a variable excess of blasts. It can be distinguished from juvenile chronic myelomonocytic leukaemia (see below) by the chromosome abnormality and lack of fetal red cell changes. The patient illustrated had a high WBC which tends to evolve as the disease progresses. The eventual transformation to acute myeloid leukaemia is the rule. The tendency to infection is at least in part due to an associated neutrophil function defect.

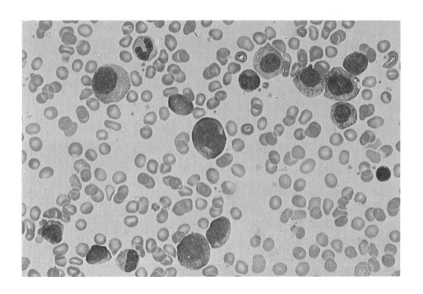

9.4 RAEB with monosomy 7
Bone marrow

An excess of blasts (8 per cent in this aspirate) with associated erythrodysplasia.

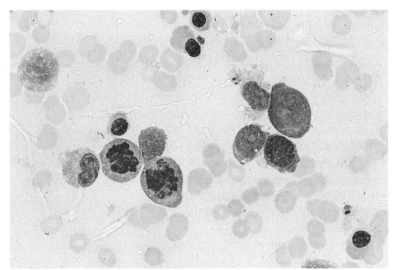

9.5 RAEB with monosomy 7
Bone marrow

As above; atypical and poorly granulated myeloid precursors.

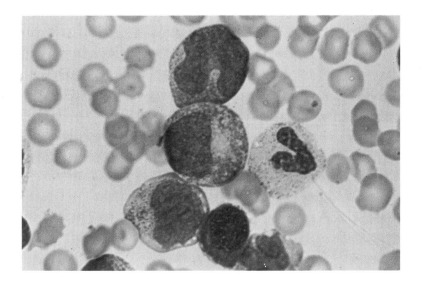

9.6 RAEB with monosomy 7
   Bone marrow
As above; eosinophils with atypical
morphology are commonly seen.

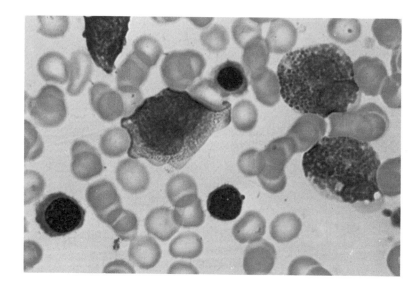

9.7 RAEB with monosomy 7
   Trephine biopsy
Boy of 5 years. Shows myeloproliferation
with mixed population.

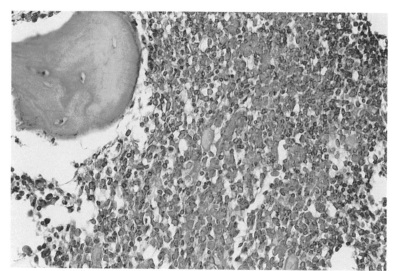

9.8 RAEB with monosomy 7
   Trephine biopsy; reticulin stain
Increased reticulin and accompanying
fibrosis are usual in this syndrome—
aspiration of marrow is often difficult.

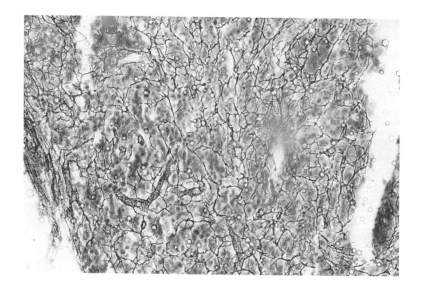

9.9   Down's syndrome—leukaemoid reaction

Trephine biopsy

Concurrent with 9.38 and 9.39 from same case. Heterogeneous cell population with no evidence of leukaemia. Cellularity unremarkable for age.

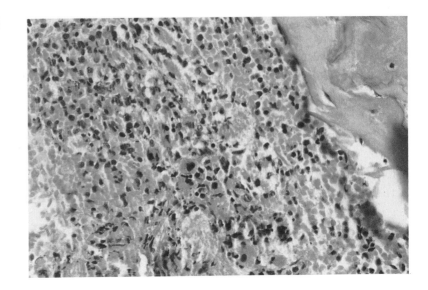

9.10   Down's syndrome— myelofibrosis/leukaemia; RAEB(T)

Blood film

Circulating blasts in a 3½-year-old simple trisomy Down syndrome girl. She had had a perinatal leukaemoid phase as above (9.9) with a WBC of $169 \times 10^9/l$, aged 4 days, which disappeared without marrow failure over 2 months. The blasts marked with CDw41 (platelet glycoprotein IIb/IIIa). They reappeared 3 years later with progressive marrow failure and fibrosis. Haemoglobin 6.6 g/dl; WBC $30.9 \times 10^9/l$; blasts 8 per cent, platelets $64 \times 10^9/l$.

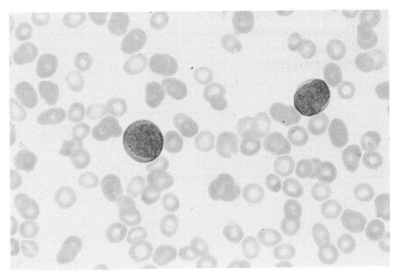

9.11   Down's syndrome— myelofibrosis/leukaemia; RAEB(T)

Bone marrow

Same case as 9.10. Marrow very difficult to aspirate; blasts 25 per cent of nucleated cells. Karyotype of marrow showed mosaicism with most cells having abnormalities additional to the trisomy 21 (48, XX, 6q−, +11, +21). Blasts appeared to be of megakaryocyte lineage. Two are seen in this frame. At this stage the syndrome would qualify for the group of myelodysplasias known as RAEB(T).

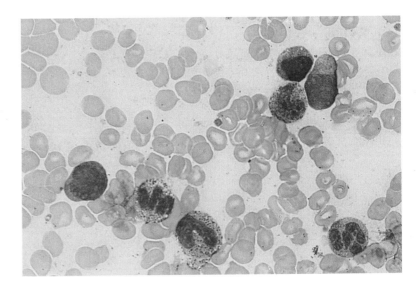

**9.12 Down's syndrome—
myelofibrosis/leukaemia;
RAEB(T)**
Trephine biopsy
Low power view showing gross
hypercellularity. Same case as 9.10.

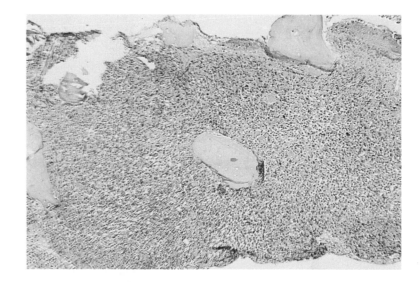

**9.13 Down's syndrome—
myelofibrosis/leukaemia;
RAEB(T)**
Trephine biopsy; reticulin stain
Increased reticulin and fibroblasts (same
case as 9.10).

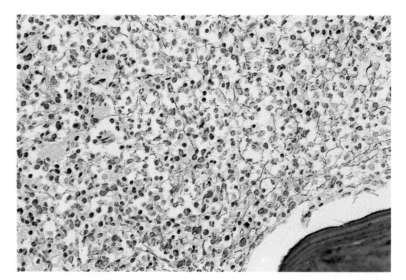

9.14 RAEB(T)
Bone marrow
A six-year-old girl with a pancytopenia
and a few circulating blast cells and
myelocytes. A rare condition in childhood
without monosomy 7 (see below), which
usually progresses to acute leukaemia.

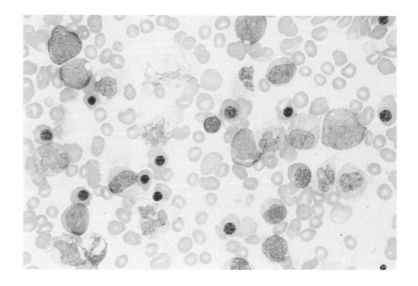

9.15   Monosomy 7 myelodysplasia
Fluorescence *in situ*
Hybridization (FISH)

The best modern test for monosomy 7 is
FISH. The normal cell on the left shows
two yellow dots on chromosome 7 and
two red dots on chromosome 22. The
abnormal cell on the right demonstrates
one missing chromosome 7. This is a
rapid and reliable test.

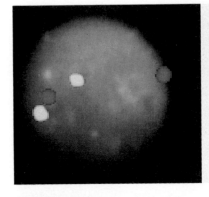
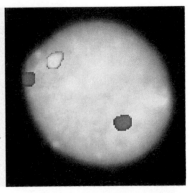

9.16   Abnormal localization of immature progenitors (ALIPS)
Bone marrow trephine

ALIPS is simply the presence of blast cells
towards the centre of the marrow cavity
and away from the trabeculae, which is
their normal position.   This is said to be
of some prognostic importance in
myelodysplasias where it is commonly
seen but this has not yet been fully
evaluated in children.

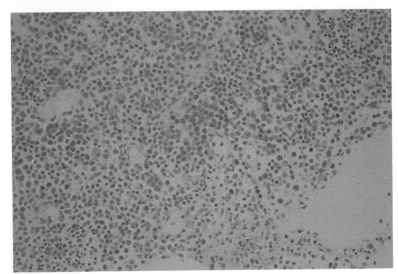

9.17   Abnormal localization of immature progenitors (ALIPS)
Marrow trephine

See 9.16. The blast cells are clearly seen to
be 'displaced' away from the trabeculae.

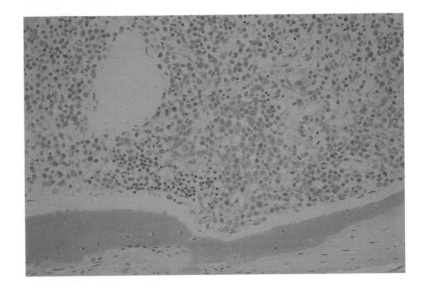

9.18 Juvenile chronic myeloid leukaemia (JCML)
Blood film

This condition is more accurately called childhood sub-acute myelomonocytic leukaemia. It arises in infants and can be distinguished from 'adult' type chronic granulocytic leukaemia (see below) by the clinical picture (lymphadenopathy, rashes, bruising); the blood findings (fetal red cell characteristics, thrombocytopenia, atypical monocytosis); and marrow cytogenetics (the Ph[1] chromosome is absent). Otherwise the two disorders can be confused. In the child illustrated, the WBC was $18 \times 10^9/l$ with 17 per cent monocytes with the morphology shown.

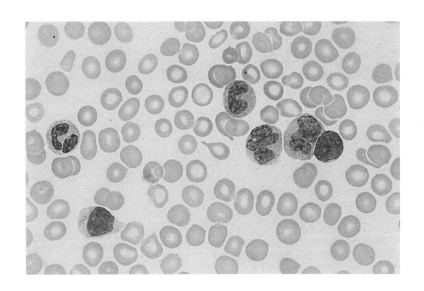

9.19 Juvenile chronic myeloid leukaemia (JCML)
Bone marrow

A mixed picture with a variable though usually modest excess of blasts.

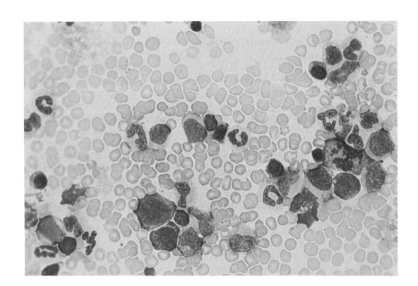

9.20 Juvenile chronic myeloid leukaemia with erythroid 'crisis'
Marrow

JCML patients have a propensity to develop a proliferation of erythroid precursors which may show dysplastic changes, as in this case. Rarely, a true erythroleukaemia (AML M6) may develop.

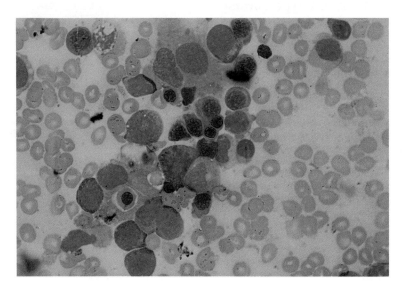

9.21   Juvenile chronic myeloid leukaemia
Trephine biopsy

Dense hypercellular marrow. Child aged 3 years.

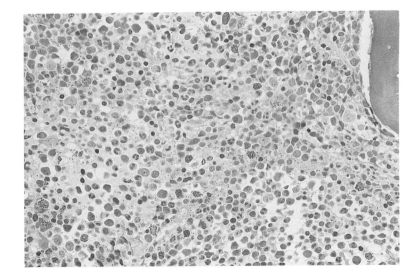

9.22   Juvenile chronic myeloid leukaemia
Blood film; Kleihauer stain

A striking characteristic of JCML is the frequently encountered high concentration of HbF with a heterogeneous distribution among the red cells as shown in this untransfused patient. Parallel fetal red cell changes seen include increased i antigen expression, and reduced carbonic anhydrase. Such features are not invariable.

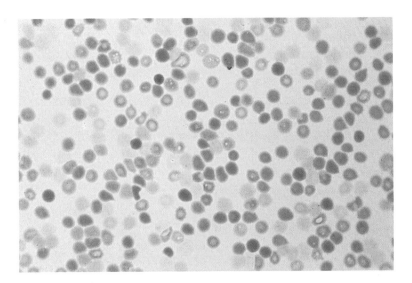

9.23   'Adult'-type chronic granulocytic leukaemia
Blood film

The disease seen in children does not differ from that seen in adults. The presenting features are similar—massive splenomegaly, gross leucocytosis sometimes sufficient to cause vascular sludging, (in the case illustrated, a 10-year-old boy, the WBC was $849 \times 10^9/l$), anaemia, and fatigue. There is usually an associated basophilia, and granulocyte alkaline phosphatase activity is low. The Ph[1] chromosome is nearly always present.

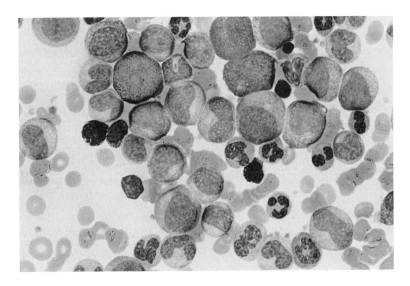

9.24 'Adult'-type chronic granulocytic leukaemia
Bone marrow
Cytology of marrow aspirates is not qualitatively abnormal in any specific way. There is little associated fibrosis, so a densely cellular aspirate is usually easily obtained.

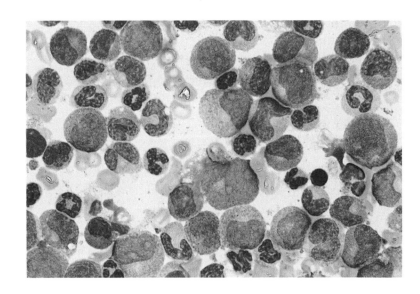

9.25 'Adult'-type chronic granulocytic leukaemia
Bone marrow
Foamy cells, shown here, and cells resembling Gaucher cells, shown below in 9.26 , are sometimes seen in a marrow giving rise to a mistaken diagnosis of a storage disorder

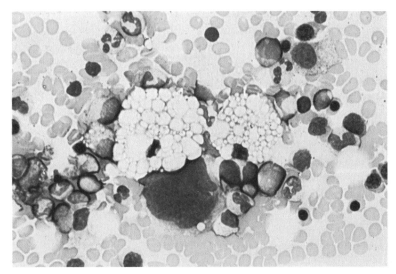

9.26 'Adult'-type chronic granulocytic leukaemia
Bone marrow
Pseudo-Gaucher cells (see also 9.25).

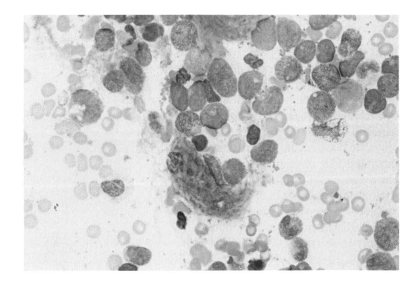

9.27 'Adult'-type chronic granulocytic leukaemia
Trephine biopsy
Myeloproliferation with total loss of fat spaces (same patient as 9.23, 9.24).

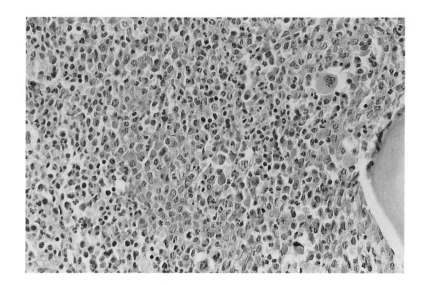

9.28 'Adult'-type chronic granulocytic leukaemia—Ph[1]-negative
Blood film
Occasional examples of Ph[1]-negative CGL (other than juvenile CML) are seen in childhood. This film is from a 9-year-old whose disease was clinically more aggressive than Ph[1]-positive CGL. She responded well to a histocompatible marrow allograft.

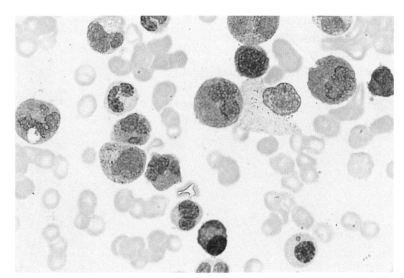

9.29 Primary myelofibrosis
Blood film
Primary myelofibrosis (agnogenic myeloid metaplasia, AMM) is an adult disorder that is very rare in childhood and any patient who might have it should be thoroughly investigated to exclude other causes of marrow fibrosis such as those above. It does occur. The patient illustrated had concomitant folate lack, which can complicate any myeloproliferative state. Tear-drop poikilocytes are seen in the case illustrated. Other features include leucoerythroblastosis, Pelger–Hüet cells and giant platelets.

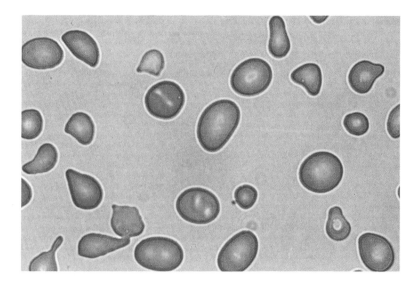

9.30 Primary myelofibrosis
Trephine biopsy; reticulin stain
This shows the typical fibrillary pattern of a myelofibrotic marrow and is taken from the patient whose blood film is shown in 9.29.

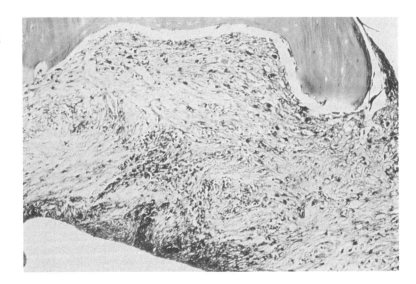

9.31 Essential thrombocythaemia
Bone marrow trephine
The trephine shows marked expansion of granulocytic and erythroid elements with abundant megakaryocytes. This rare myeloproliferative disorder of childhood affected a 4-year-old girl who presented with peripheral vascular insufficiency and a platelet count of $1000 \times 10^9/l$.

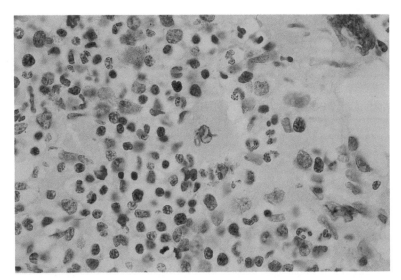

9.32 Polycythaemia
Bone marrow trephine
By far the commonest causes of a high red cell count in childhood are cardiopulmonary disorders and dehydration. Very rarely it can be due to an abnormal high-affinity haemoglobin. Other cases can be secondary to erythropoietin-secreting tumours of the posterior cranial fossa, kidney, and liver. Others, as in this case, are due to high erythropoietin of unknown aetiology. The trephine shows marked expansion of the erythroid and megakaryocyte series.

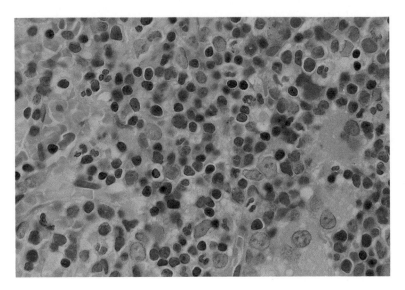

9.33   Hypereosinophilic syndrome due to t;5:12
Blood film

This adolescent boy has a long history of a dramatic urticarial rash. The blood, marrow, and skin biopsies all show eosinophilia. Other cases have been described in which lung infiltrates (Löeffler's syndrome) and tricuspid valve incompetence occur, secondary to eosinophil infiltration. However, the commonest causes of eosinophilia are atopy, parasites, and drugs.

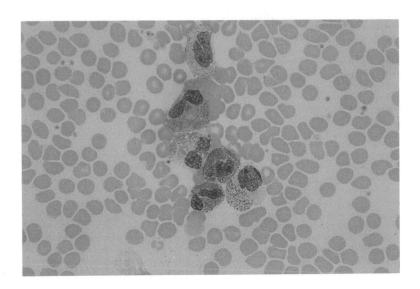

9.34   Hypereosinophilic syndrome due to t;5:12
Bone marrow

The chromosomal translocation in this case involves the area coding for the IL-5 gene, suggesting that there is aberrant production of this cytokine which controls eosinophils.

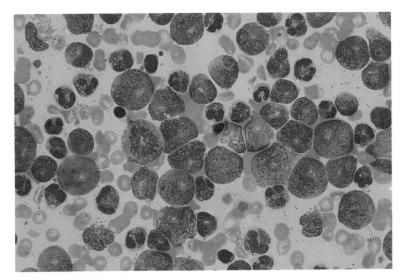

9.35   Pearson's syndrome (bone marrow-pancreas syndrome)
Blood film

A 5-month-old girl presented with severe anaemia which became transfusion dependent. The anaemia was normocytic and normochromic although it can be macrocytic in Pearson's syndrome. Pearson's syndrome is a mitochondrial cytopathy with mitochondrial DNA deletions and is confirmed by DNA analysis (Southern blotting). Other tissues are involved, in particular pancreas, liver, and the central nervous system. Sixty percent of patients die of organ dysfunction within 3 years of diagnosis but the blood disorder sometimes improves and may proceed to Kearns–Sayre syndrome if survival permits.

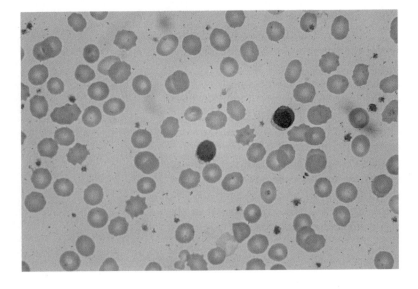

9.36 Pearson's syndrome
Bone marrow

The same patient as in 9.35. Siderotic granules are present in the late normoblast and prominent vacuoles in the proerythroblast. These features, along with ringed sideroblasts, are distinctive features of this syndrome, but may also be seen in myelodysplastic syndromes. However, Pearson's syndrome must be considered in all cases of sideroblastic anaemia in early childhood.

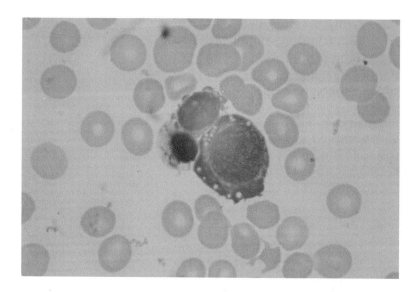

9.37 Pearson's syndrome
Bone marrow; Perls' Stain

The vacuolation is seen, along with a ringed sideroblast.

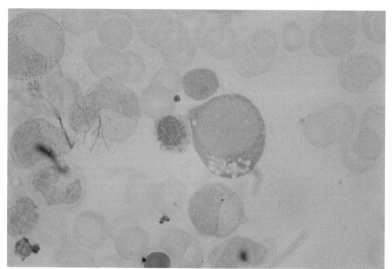

9.38 Down's syndrome. Transient abnormal myelopoiesis (TAM)
Blood film

Film from a 3-day-old simple trisomy Down's syndrome baby showing blast cells. His WBC was $44 \times 10^9/l$ (37 per cent blasts); haemoglobin 24.7 g/dl; platelets $120 \times 10^9/l$. The marrow is shown in 9.39. The blasts disappeared by the age of 3 months and bone marrow failure never occurred. The boy remains well 5 years later.

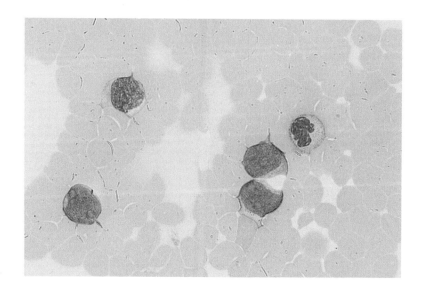

9.39   Down's syndrome. Transient abnormal myelopoiesis (TAM)
Blood film

Marrow aspirate from same case as 9.38 concurrent with blood film. Blasts comprised only 18 per cent of the total nucleated cells. Karyotype on bone marrow showed simple trisomy 21. The blasts appeared myeloid in origin. No megakaryocyte markers were seen.

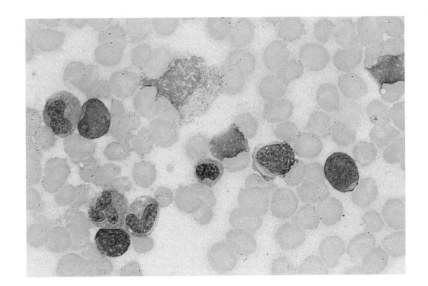

10
Histiocyte–monocyte disorders

Classification of histiocytosis syndromes

(after Histiocyte Society Classification: *Lancet* (1987), **1**, 208–9.)

Class I   Langerhans cell histiocytosis (LCH)

(Formerly 'histiocytosis X' and including 'eosinophilic granuloma', 'Hand–Schüller–Christian disease', and 'Letterer–Siwe disease'.)

Class II   'Non-malignant' histiocytosis of mononuclear phagocytes other than Langerhans cells

(a)   Haemophagocytic lymphohistiocytosis (HLH)
  (i)   *genetic/familial* (F-HLH): (formerly 'familial erythrophagocytic lymphohistiocytosis')
  (ii) *sporadic* (formerly 'virus-associated haemophagocytic syndrome (VAHS)' or 'infection-associated haemophagocytic syndrome (IAHS)')
(b)   Other histiocytoses
  (i)   Rosai–Dorfman disease
  (ii) Xanthogranuloma
  (iii) Reticulohistiocytoma

Class III   Malignant histiocytosis

(a)   Acute monocytic leukaemia (FAB M5)
(b)   Malignant histiocytosis

Notes:
(i)   For a wide-ranging discussion of Langerhans cell histiocytosis see Special Supplement XXIII of the *Brit. J. Cancer*, **70**, (1994).
(ii) The disorders listed under Class II (b)—'other' histiocytoses—are usually clinically localized and are hardly ever organ- or life-threatening. There is therefore a case for moving them to a 'new' Class IV (see Pritchard, J. and Broadbent, V. (1994). *Brit. J. Canc.*, **70**, S1–S3.)
(iii) Malignant histiocytosis (MH) is exceedingly rare in children. Until the mid-1980s many cases of 'large cell NHL' were mistakenly labelled 'malignant histiocytosis' but, because of widespread use of modern immunohistochemical analysis especially the Ki-1 antibody, such errors are now rare.

Acute monocytic leukaemia is dealt with in Chapter 8 of this volume, but is also included in this classification to remind readers of the overlap between the non-lymphoblastic acute leukaemia and the histiocyte–monocyte disorders.

10.1   Langerhans cell histiocytosis
Bone marrow

This 2-year-old boy had marked hepatosplenomegaly, disseminated bone disease, and a rash.

The changes in the bone marrow in 'LCH' are variable and, without special stains, not diagnostic. In many cases large foamy histiocytes are found in marrow aspirates. In other instances the histiocytes may be less mature looking, can resemble those found in skin and other tissue biopsies and may be CD1a positive ('LCH cells'). Marrow infiltration *per se*, even with CD1a-positive cells, does not necessarily indicate a poor prognosis.

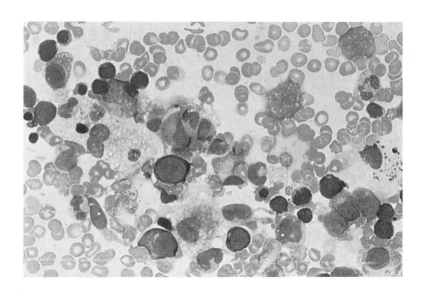

10.2   Langerhans cell histiocytosis
Bone marrow trephine; plastic section

The morphology of the 'LCH cells' is better seen than in paraffin sections and the typical folded nucleus and reniform nuclear shapes are readily appreciated.

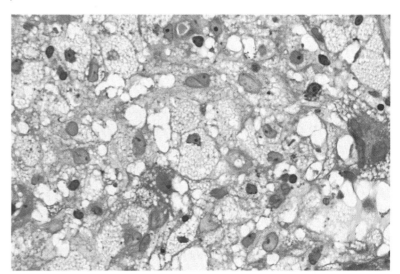

10.3   Langerhans cell histiocytosis
Bone marrow

This infant had progressive life-threatening disease with evidence of liver failure (hypoproteinaemia and abnormal coagulation). The marrow contains many cells with long processes. Though striking, this appearance is still not diagnostic without specific 'marker' studies (see 10.4 and 10.5).

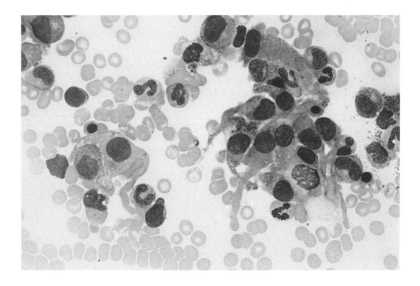

10.4 Langerhans cell histiocytosis
Bone marrow; α-mannosidase activity

The cells with long processes (see 10.3) exhibit intense focal α-mannosidase activity characteristic of 'LCH cells'. Some 'rounded' histiocytes are also present and also show intense focal α-mannosidase activity. Normal marrow cells, by contrast, have only weak diffuse activity. Although more or less specific for 'LCH cells' this reaction is difficult to perform and anti CD1a staining is usually now preferred.

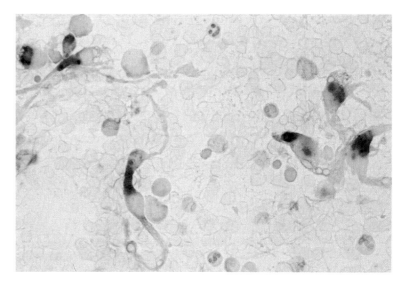

10.5 Langerhans cell histiocytosis
Bone marrow; CD1a stain

In this child with bone marrow involvement, positive CD1a staining (APAAP technique) is evident in the left-hand panel. This stain, and the identification of Birbeck granules by electron microscopy (10.6), are the most 'definitive' laboratory investigations for 'LCH cells'. In the right-hand panel a foamy ordinary histiocyte is CD1a-negative. While S100 protein and peanut agglutinin are important markers for LCH in skin, they are unhelpful and non-specific in marrow.

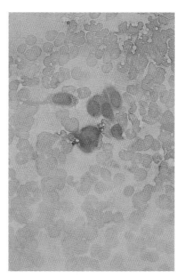 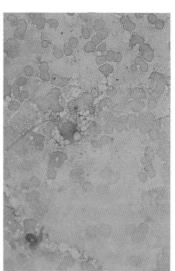

10.6 Langerhans cell histiocytosis
Electron photomicrograph

The striking appearance of the Birbeck granules (single arrows) identifies the probable Langerhans cell origin of 'LCH cells'. Tennis racquet-like forms (double arrow) may also be seen and granules cut in cross-section may be ring-like or target-like. The Birbeck granules may not be found without a considerable search and up to 30 potential 'LCH cells' may need to be examined.

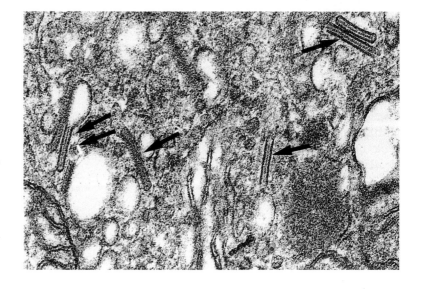

10.7   Langerhans cell histiocytosis
Bone marrow

Secondary erythrophagocytosis, while said to be rare, is actually quite common in bone-marrow aspirates in Langerhans cell histiocytosis. As shown in this illustration it is the ordinary (phagocytic) foamy histiocytes, which are CD1a negative, that engulf other bone marrow cells. CD1a-positive 'LCH cells' are non-phagocytic.

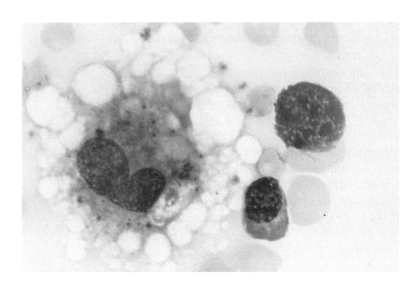

10.8   Langerhans cell histiocytosis
Bone marrow; iron stain

The presence of iron in macrophages indicates that a marked degree of erythrophagocytosis has taken place. However, erythrophagocytosis is a very non-specific phenomenon and occurs in many conditions ranging from Langerhans cell histiocytosis and HLH to post-transfusion states and 'auto-immune' disorders (see 10.17), T-cell lymphoma, rhabdomyosarcoma, and various other malignant tumours. Minor degrees of haemophagocytosis can even be found in ostensibly 'normal' bone marrow aspirates.

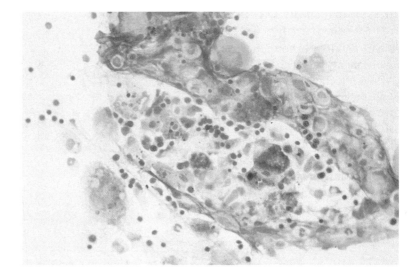

10.9   Langerhans cell histiocytosis
Lymph node; touch preparation

As shown here the morphology of histiocytes in this disorder can vary considerably and often includes multinucleate forms. As in the case of bone marrow (and other tissues), definitive diagnosis of LCH cannot be made unless either Birbeck granules are identified (see 10.6) or CD1a staining (see 10.5) is positive.

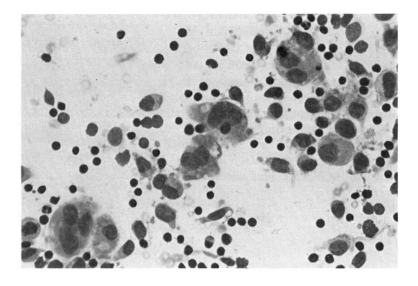

10.10 Haemophagocytic lymphohistiocytosis (familial/ genetic form)
Lymph node; H&E

This section shows many large macrophages full of ingested red cells. The patient presented (typically) at the age of 6 months with pancytopenia, fever, and hepatosplenomegaly with jaundice. Lymph node and liver biopsy, as well as bone-marrow aspirate, revealed erythrophagocytosis. The patient had a sibling who had died with a similar disorder. The degree of erythrophagocytosis in the marrow varies a great deal and repeated sampling or liver biopsy may be needed (though coagulopathy may make these procedures risky).

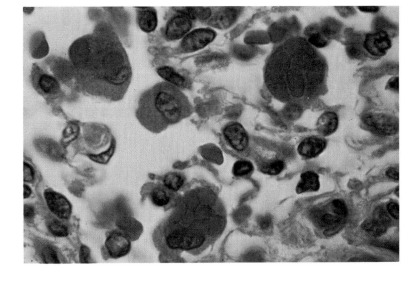

10.11 Haemophagocytic lymphohistiocytosis (familial/ genetic form)
Lymph node; touch preparation

This shows two phagocytic histiocytes full of ingested red cells and some platelets. The clinical picture was similar to that of the child whose biopsy is shown in 10.10. The diagnosis of HLH (familial type) is made by the combination of clinical features and positive family history, associated with findings of high plasma triglyceride levels and abnormally long coagulation times. CNS involvement is common.

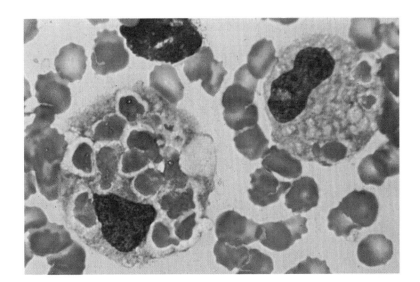

10.12 Haemophagocytic lymphohistiocytosis—sporadic
Bone marrow

This patient, aged 11 years, presented with recurrent fever, hepatosplenomegaly, and pancytopenia. Erythrophagocytosis is easily seen. The presence of haemophagocytosis is not itself diagnostic (see 10.8). However, in this case, the patient's age makes it very likely that the HLH is 'sporadic' and an infectious agent may be identified. In 'sporadic' HLH, or in the genetic form, the CSF may be abnormal and phagocytosis by mononuclear cells may be seen.

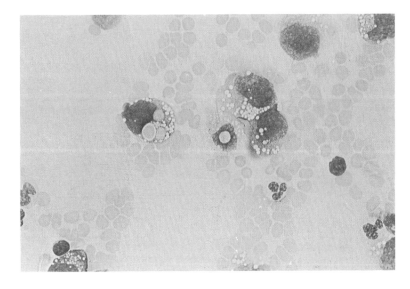

10.13   Haemophagocytic lymphohistiocytosis
Bone marrow

Red cells, a normoblast, and a neutrophil have been ingested by a phagocytic histiocyte. It is unlikely that red cells are more 'tasty' to phagocytic cells than platelets or white cells—there are simply more of them in the circulating blood.

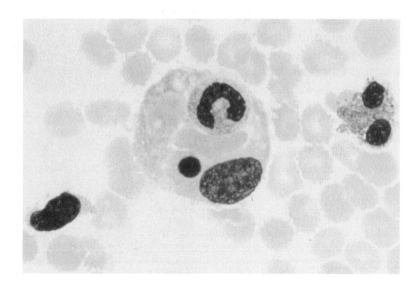

10.14   Haemophagocytic lymphohistiocytosis
Bone marrow

Platelets can also be ingested by phagocytic histiocytes.

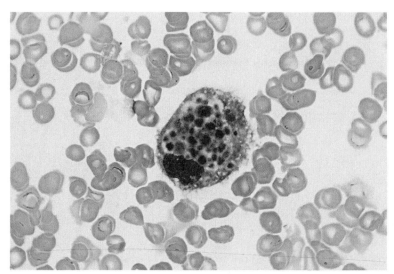

10.15   Haemophagocytic lymphohistiocytosis
Cerebrospinal fluid

Phagocytosis (in this case of platelets) by mononuclear cells is a frequent but not invariable finding, both in 'familial/genetic' and 'sporadic' HLH. Patients with a 'positive' CSF may have signs of CNS malfunction, especially fits and/or encephalopathy. With CNS involvement there is often a raised cell count in the CSF.

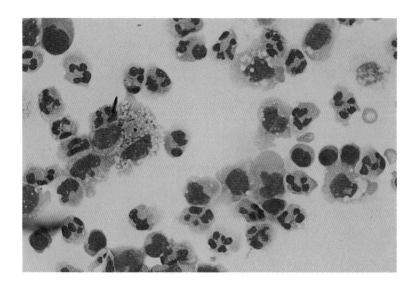

10.16 Haemophagocytic lymphohistiocytosis
Bone-marrow aspirate

In 'end-stage' HLH (familial/genetic or sporadic) the marrow may become aplastic, presumably because of either haemophagocytosis of bone marrow stem cells, or cytokine induced damage, or both mechanisms.

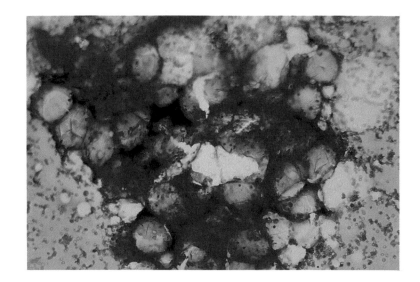

10.17 Secondary haemophagocytosis
Bone marrow

In this composite picture histiocytes are seen ingesting red cells, debris, and nuclear material. The sample is from a 12-year-old boy who was later diagnosed as having dermatomyositis. The haemophagocytosis was presumably immune-mediated in this instance. The illustrations re-emphasize that haemophagocytosis is a microscope appearance and *not* a 'diagnosis' in itself.

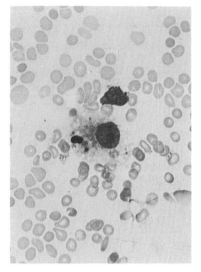 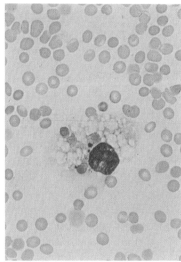

11
Lymphomas

11.1 Normal lymph node
Touch preparation
The appearances of a normal lymph node are shown. The cut surface of the node is lightly pressed on to a glass slide and the imprint is fixed and stained. Lymphocytes are heterogeneous and scattered macrophages are seen.

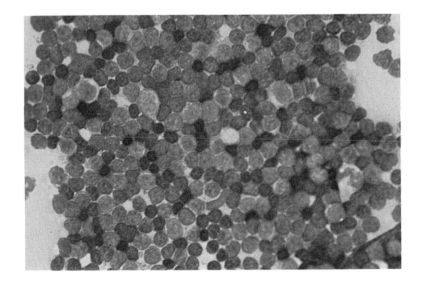

11.2 Non-Hodgkin's lymphoma
Lymph node; touch preparation
Compare with 11.1. There is a more homogeneous population of large blast cells, but normal appearances may vary especially in reactive nodes, and a confident diagnosis should not be made without histopathology and immunocytochemistry.

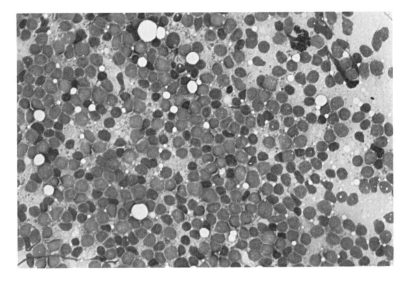

11.3 B-lymphoblastic lymphoma (Burkitt type)
Lymph node; touch preparation

This plate shows sheets of vacuolated blasts with interspersed macrophages. This so-called 'starry sky' appearance is not specific and is seen in other lymphomas. The B-cell origin of this tumour was confirmed by immunocytochemistry.

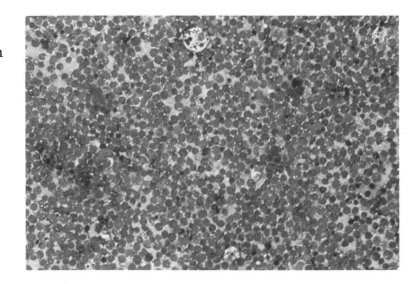

11.4 Normal lymph nodes
Touch preparation; acid phosphatase

Some block positivity of T-cells and strong diffuse positivity of macrophages is shown.

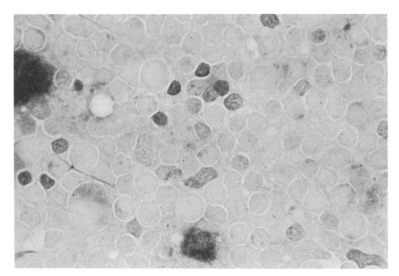

11.5 Non-Hodgkin's lymphoma
Touch preparation; acid phosphatase

This preparation (same case as 11.2) shows striking block positivity in most cells. A T-lymphoblastic lymphoma was confirmed by immunocytochemistry.

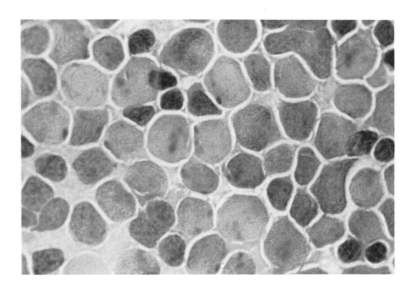

11.6   Hodgkin's lymphoma

Lymph node; touch preparation
A classical Reed–Sternberg cell with
double nucleoli and 'owl's eye' nucleoli is
shown.

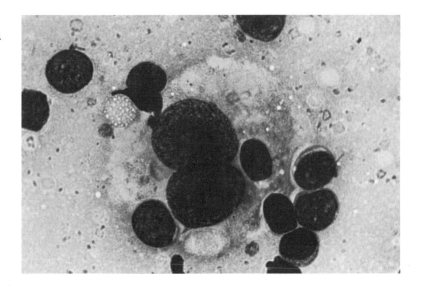

11.7   Hodgkin's lymphoma

Bone marrow trephine; HE
This 8-year-old girl presented with fever
and splenomegaly. There is a dense
fibrosis evident at low power. An increase
in reticulin may be the only evidence of
Hodgkin's lymphoma in bone marrow,
and along with an eosinophilia should
make one suspicious of this diagnosis in
this clinical setting.

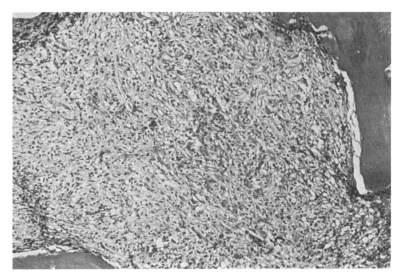

11.8   Hodgkin's lymphoma; pre-treatment

Bone marrow trephine; reticulin
This stain of the same sample shown in
11.7 clearly demonstrates the fibrosis
commonly present when Hodgkin's
lymphoma involves the marrow. Secondary
myelofibrosis may also be present without
overt tumour invasion.

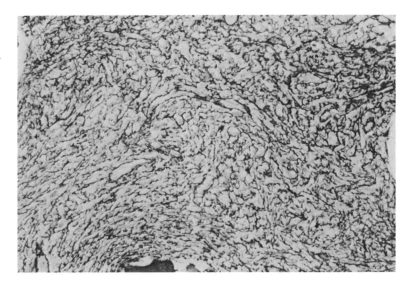

11.9 Hodgkin's lymphoma; after chemotherapy

Bone marrow trephine; reticulin
Just after the trephine biopsy shown in 11.8 was taken, the patient was treated with quadruple chemotherapy. Six months later she was in complete remission and the bone marrow trephine showed no evidence of fibrosis.

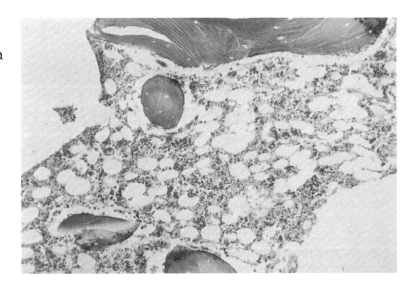

11.10 Large cell anaplastic lymphoma Ki-1 positive (CD30)

Bone marrow
Ki-1 lymphoma typically involves lymph nodes and often skin, lung, and other peripheral sites. The CNS is infrequently affected but the marrow is infiltrated in Stage IV cases. The presence of circulating lymphoma cells is rare. Diagnosis can be difficult because of its protean manifestations, including PUO.

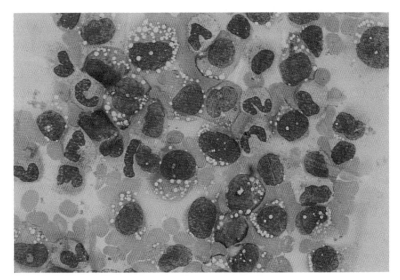

12

Other tumours: small round cell tumours of childhood involving the bone marrow

Although other types of cancer (such as Hodgkin's disease) sometimes infiltrate the bone marrow, the most common problem in differential diagnosis is the distinction between the so-called 'small round cell tumours of childhood'. A working classification is listed below, in approximate descending order of frequency. Acute leukaemias are included both because they *are* 'small round cell tumours' and also because there may be genuine difficulty in distinguishing between acute leukaemia, when the peripheral blood is normal, and a 'solid' tumour involving the bone marrow. Alongside the classification are listed the most common chromosome abnormality occurring in each type of tumour cell. These genetic anomalies are now of major practical importance because of the increasing use of *in situ* hybridization, especially 'FISH' (fluorescent *in situ* hybridization), in tumour diagnosis. Examples are shown in plates 12.10–12.12 and 12.21.

Tumour type	Chromosome abnormality in tumour cell
Acute leukaemia	Various[1]
Non-Hodgkin's lymphoma	
Neuroblastoma	1p3.1–1p3.6 del
	N myc amplification
Rhabdomyosarcoma (alveolar subtype)	t2q:13q
Primitive neuro-ectodermal tumour (PNET)[2] including Ewing's tumour	t11q:22q
Retinoblastoma	13q del

[1] Each 'FAB' subtype of ALL and ANLL has one or more characteristic chromosome changes, too numerous to list here (but see sections, 7, 8, and 11).

[2] 'Peripheral' PNET is a tumour occurring in many parts of the body outside the CNS. The term 'central' PNET denotes a primitive neuro-ectodermal tumour arising within the central nervous system (CNS). These tumours should be distinguished from 'peripheral PNETs' which, despite a neural origin and the similar (confusing) names, 'central' and 'peripheral' PNETs are probably completely different tumour types. In particular, the t11q:22q translocation characteristic of 'peripheral' PNET, including Ewing's tumour, has never been described in 'central' PNET. Ewing's tumour is now regarded by most people as a 'peripheral PNET' arising in bone.

'Central' PNET, which rarely if ever appears in bone, includes all tumours currently identified by their anatomical location—medulloblastoma, pinealoblastoma, and supratentorial PNET. Ependymoma is not, strictly speaking, a 'small round cell tumour' but the 'ependymoblastoma', which usually occurs in infancy, may have this appearance.

12.1   Small round cell tumour of childhood

Touch preparation; marrow trephine

Clumps of tumour cells are seen with free tumour cells in the surrounding areas. Accurate diagnosis of small round cell tumours is not possible from bone-marrow aspirates alone. Plastic sections of trephines, to give better morphology, will help but tissue diagnosis, supplemented by immunohistochemical studies, is essential.

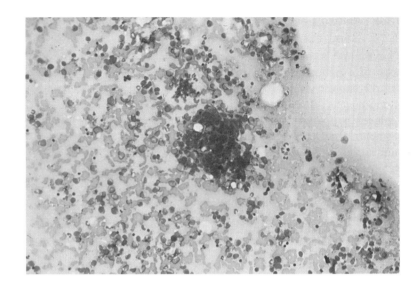

12.2   Small round cell tumour of childhood

Touch preparation; marrow trephine

Clumps of tumour cells, showing vacuolation, are seen under high-power examination. Distinction between solid tumours is impossible in this type of preparation, but, especially when the primary tumour cannot be identified or biopsied, FISH studies on bone marrow may be crucial.

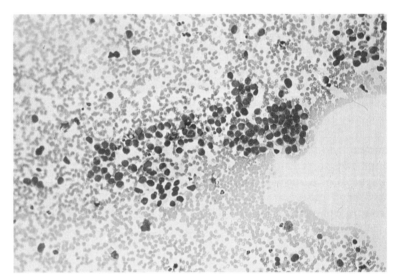

12.3   Neuroblastoma

Bone marrow

A 3-year-old boy presented with anaemia and bone pain. Abdominal ultrasound examination revealed a right adrenal mass and the urinary HVA/VMA excretion were significantly elevated.

This plate shows a clump of tumour cells in an otherwise normal marrow.

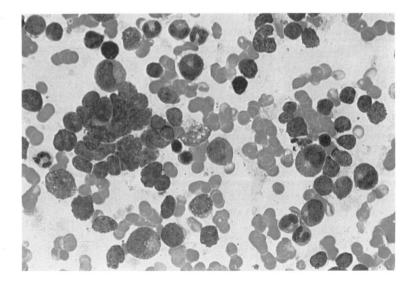

12.4   Neuroblastoma
Bone marrow

This sample is taken from the right iliac crest of a patient whose left iliac crest sample showed only rare, equivocal 'tumour cells'. This marrow is almost replaced by malignant cells forming sheets ('syncitia') rather than rosettes. Marrow infiltration by neuroblastoma may be patchy and trephine biopsy is essential when this diagnosis or a diagnosis of any other marrow-infiltrating tumour is suspected.

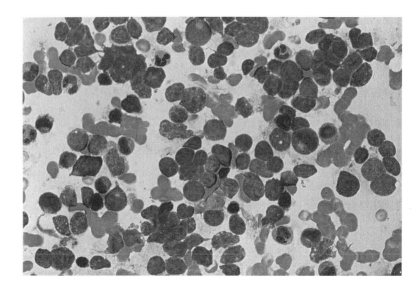

12.5   Neuroblastoma
Bone marrow

High-power view of a clump of tumour cells. The cells can usually be distinguished from lymphoma/leukaemia cells by their patchy distribution, their tendency to clump and form 'syncitia', and by their relatively low nuclear:cytoplasmic ratio. However, it is important to re-emphasize that the diagnosis of a specific small round cell tumour in bone marrow cannot be made from morphology alone.

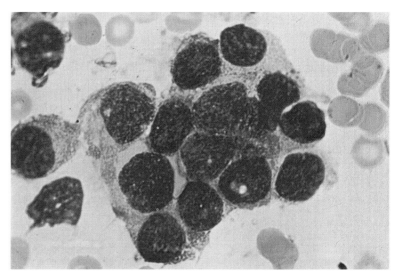

12.6   Neuroblastoma
Bone marrow

This shows near-complete replacement of marrow by vacuolated tumour cells. The patient, aged 18 months, had a large adrenal mass. The clinical picture, with cell surface marker studies (see 12.7), and raised concentrations of urinary VMA and HVA gave the diagnosis, which was confirmed on the resected primary tumour. Vacuolation may also be seen in other childhood cancer cells, e.g. rhabdomyosarcoma (12.22) and Ewing's tumour (12.17) and acute leukaemia, especially in the M4-5 and L3 FAB subtypes.

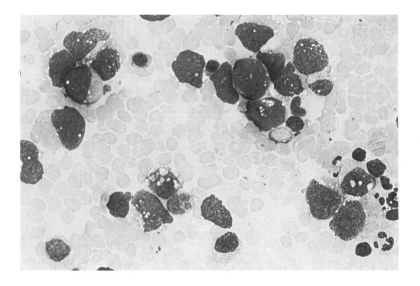

12.7 Neuroblastoma
Bone marrow

A group of tumour cells is detected by fluorescein-labelled antibody UJ13A (left) among the cluster of cells seen by phase-contrast microscopy (right). Care is needed in the interpretation of preparations stained with this antibody as it is known to cross-react with osteoblasts (Roald, B. and Kemshead, J., personal communication).

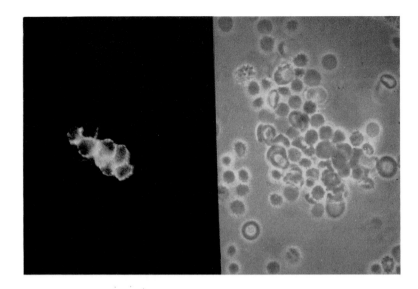

12.8 Neuroblastoma
Bone marrow trephine; plastic section

Thin sections of resin-embedded trephines offer much better morphology and cytological detail than paraffin sections. Malignant cells with prominent nucleoli are readily identified in this plate.

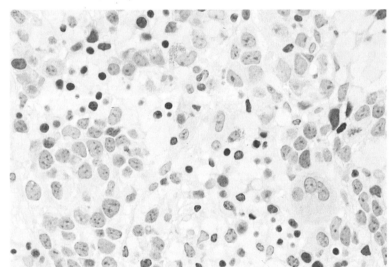

12.9 Neuroblastoma
Pleural fluid; cytocentrifuge

This cytospin deposit from a pleural effusion contains tumour cells (a) surrounded by lymphocytes (b), and macrophages (c). See accompanying diagram for the identification of the cells. It may be difficult to distinguish normal reactive mesothelial cells and malignant cells in an effusion. Therefore, diagnosis should not be based on morphology alone, but confirmed by immunohistochemical or cytogenetic techniques.

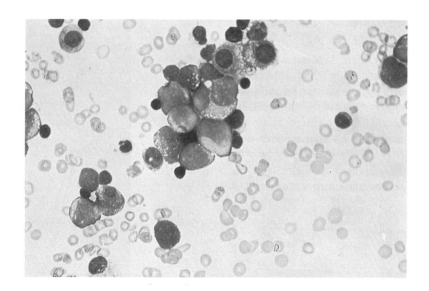

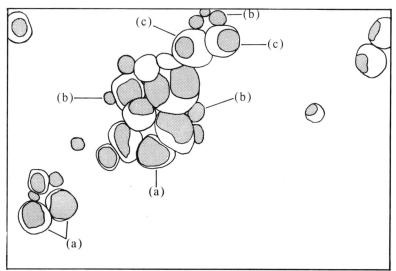

12.10 Neuroblastoma
Lymph node; fluorescent *in situ* hybridization (FISH)

The plate shows an imprint (touch preparation) from the lymph node of a child with proven stage 4 neuroblastoma. The fluorochrome-labelled N myc-specific DNA probe hybridizes to multiple copies (yellow dots) of the N myc gene sequence. Normal cells have only one copy of N myc on each chromosome 2, as seen in the lymphocyte on the right, but the gene is grossly amplified in these tumour cells. The largest cell may be tetraploid, compared with the diploid or near-diploid pair of tumour cells above it.
Amplification is, generally speaking, an 'unfavourable' prognostic feature.

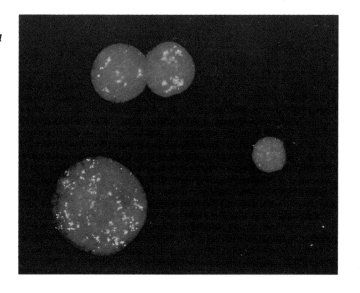

12.11 Neuroblastoma
Tumour imprints: FISH for ploidy (DNA index)

These primary neuroblastoma cells have been tested with a DNA probe specific for the centromere of chromosome 8. Although there is heterogeneity, there is clearly a triploid population of cells (three yellow dots per cell). Triploid tumours are thought to have a relatively 'favourable' prognosis compared with diploid/pseudo-diploid and tetraploid tumours.

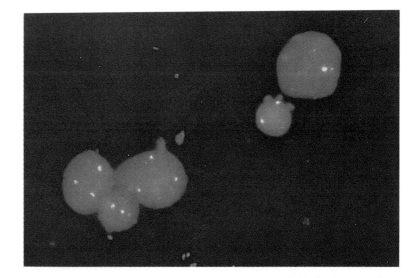

12.12 Neuroblastoma
Bone marrow; FISH

This 3-year-old child had stage 4 neuroblastoma, with metastases in bone and bone marrow and an abdominal primary tumour. The cells have been tested with a DNA probe specific for the 1p3.3 region of chromosome 1 (see introduction to this section). All the tumour cells show a single signal indicating deletion of a segment of 1p, a feature generally considered to have 'unfavourable' prognostic significance.

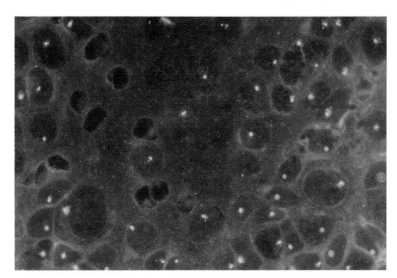

12.13 Neuroblastoma stage 4, restaging
Bone marrow trephine low-power

At first glance, this bone marrow seems heavily infiltrated by malignant tumour cells but see 12.14.

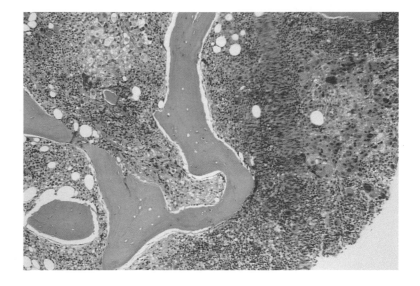

12.14 Neuroblastoma stage 4, restaging
Bone marrow trephine
This 3-year-old girl had an abdominal primary tumour with bone and bone marrow metastases. She had a good clinical response to induction chemotherapy but tumour cells persisted in the bone marrow. After 10 courses of treatment (OPEC) this bone-marrow trephine showed that many of the remaining tumour cells had 'matured' into ganglion-like cells. This phenomenon is not as well documented as 'maturation' in the primary tumour following chemotherapy and its prognostic significance is uncertain.

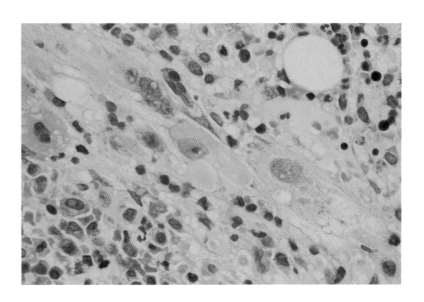

12.15 Neuroblastoma, stage 4; restaging
Bone marrow trephine, immunohistochemistry with PGP 9.5
Same case as in 12.14. The ganglionic differentiation and metastatic neuroblastoma is highlighted using the antibody PGP 9.5 which is selective for neural cells.

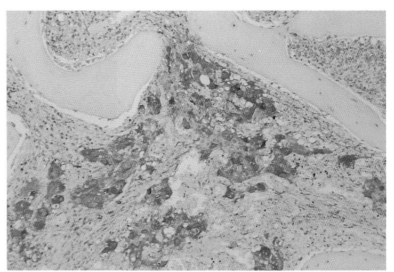

12.16 Neuroblastoma, stage 4; restaging
Bone marrow trephine, immunohistochemistry with neurofilament antibody
Same case as in 12.14. Neurofilaments (axons) are evident in this marrow trephine, not only close to the metastatic neuroblastoma deposit but also in other areas.

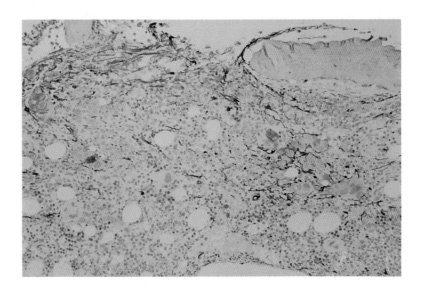

12.17 Ewing's tumour (primitive neuroectodermal tumour (PNET) of bone)
Bone marrow

A primary osteolytic tumour was present in the pelvis. There is a heavy infiltrate of mostly vacuolated tumour cells. This high-power view shows a clump of five tumour cells, two separate tumour cells, a smear cell, and a lymphocyte. There are no specific features to distinguish Ewing's tumour from other 'small cell tumours of childhood'.

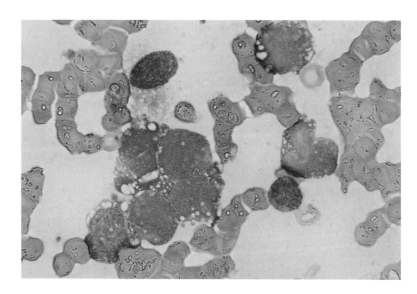

12.18 Ewing's tumour (PNET of bone)
Bone marrow; PAS

The tumour cells contain 'blocks' of PAS-positive material. The neutrophil, diffusely PAS-positive, is also present. Many tumour cell types contain glycogen and this stain is not diagnostic.

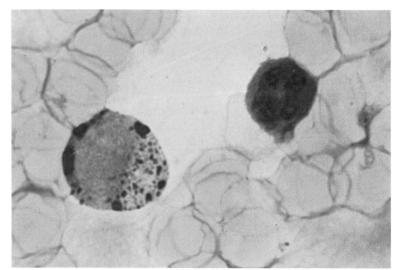

12.19 Peripheral primitive neuroectodermal tumour (PNET/Askin tumour/Ewing's tumour)
Rib biopsy

A clump of small round tumour cells in the marrow space, showing no features to distinguish them from other small round cell tumours.

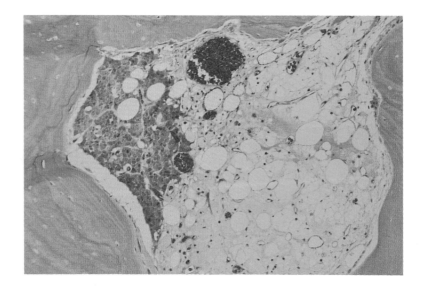

12.20 Peripheral primitive neuroectodermal tumour (PNET/Askin tumour/Ewing's tumour)

Rib biopsy; immunostaining for MIC2 gene product

The tumour cells show marked membrane staining. In the context of small round cell tumours of childhood, this pattern is indicative of PNET. Some T-cell lymphomas also express this gene product.

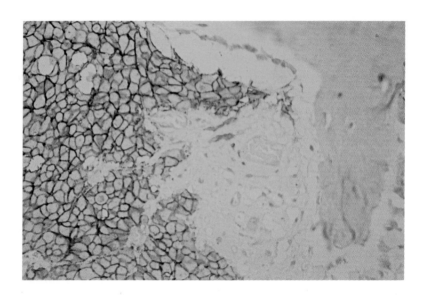

12.21 Peripheral primitive neuroectodermal tumour of soft tissue (PNET)

Tumour imprint; FISH

This 10-year-old boy had a tumour arising in the region of the olfactory plate. Tumour imprints were taken and 'two-colour FISH' carried out using probes on either side of the 11q:22q translocation characteristic of 'peripheral' PNETs. The yellow/white probe represents DNA on the centromeric side of the site of the translocation on chromosome 22, while the red probe is on the distal side of the breakpoint. On one chromosome, the two 'signals' are close together indicating a normal arrangement, but the other two 'signals' are widely separated, indicating a 11q;22q translocation.

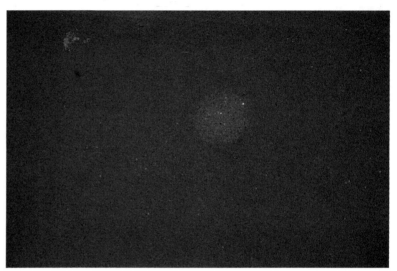

12.22 Rhabdomyosarcoma

Touch preparation of marrow trephine

A clump of tumour cells with cytoplasmic vacuolation is seen. Accurate diagnosis is not possible without further investigation as similar vacuolation may also be seen in several other types of solid tumour as well as leukaemia and lymphoma. The PAS stain for glycogen (see 12.24) is often positive in rhabdomyosarcoma but non-specific.

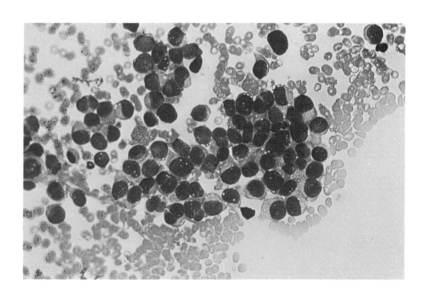

12.23 Rhabdomyosarcoma
Bone marrow

In this case the tumour cells show marked vacuolation.

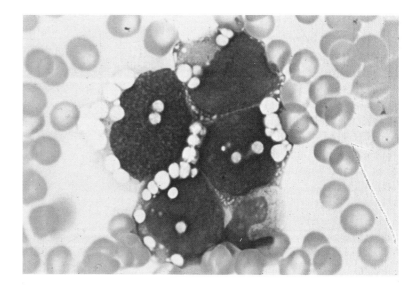

12.24 Rhabdomyosarcoma
Bone marrow PAS

The tumour cells contain masses of PAS positive blocks. A similar pattern may be seen in Ewing's tumour (see 12.18) and in acute lymphoblastic (L1 and L2) leukaemia.

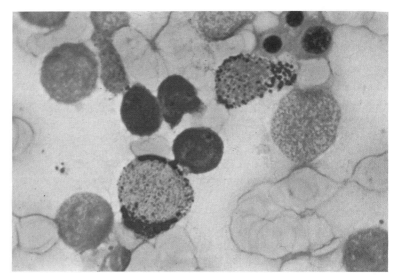

12.25 Rhabdomyosarcoma
Bone marrow trephine HE

The tumour cells have pale nuclei and are spindle-shaped but are effectively camouflaged within normal haematopoietic tissue tissue on low-power viewing.

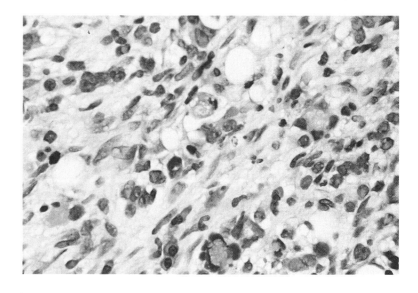

12.26 Rhabdomyosarcoma
Bone marrow trephine; immunocytochemical demonstration of desmin

The presence of desmin (yellow–brown) within the tumour cells indicates a myogenic origin and confirms the diagnosis of rhabdomyosarcoma. Other small round cell tumours are usually either desmin negative or only weakly positive.

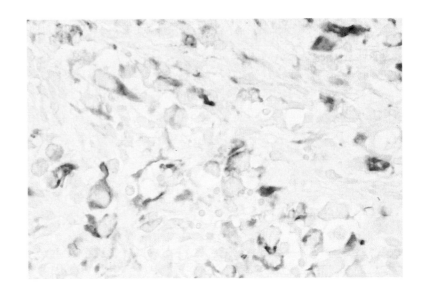

12.27 Medulloblastoma
Bone marrow

A 4-year-old child presented with acute onset of hydrocephalus, ataxia, and bone pain. Craniotomy confirmed a posterior fossa tumour. The histopathological diagnosis was medulloblastoma. Spinal MRI scans showed multiple tumour deposits. Because of bone pain, bone marrow aspirates were also carried out and tumour involvement demonstrated. This plate shows a large clump (syncitium) of tumour cells. They seem to be non-haemopoeitic but specific diagnosis is only possible when the primary tumour has been identified and/or biopsied. Bone marrow involvement is probably no more common after ventriculo-atrial or ventriculo-peritoneal shunt placement than in patients who have no shunt.

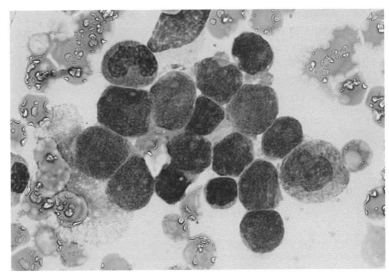

12.28 Medulloblastoma
Bone marrow trephine; HE

There is infiltration by tumour cells with some remaining normal marrow activity. In other areas there was extension of tumour into vascular spaces and marked reactive fibrosis. The bone felt abnormally hard on biopsy and no aspirate was obtained. This 14-year-old girl had no ventriculosystemic shunt.

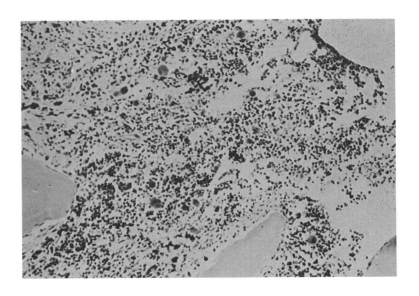

12.29 Retinoblastoma
Bone marrow

This 5-year-old boy had had treatment for a large right primary retinoblastoma three years before he presented with anaemia and bone pain. An isotope bone scan showed multiple bony metastases and the bone marrow, shown here, shows heavy infiltration by 'small round cells'. There are no features to distinguish these tumour cells from other 'small round cell tumours' of childhood.

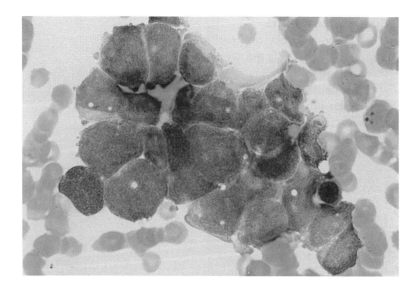

12.30 Malignant germ cell tumour: seminoma with yolk sac elements
Bone marrow trephine

A 12-year-old boy presented with leucoerythroblastic anaemia, bone pain, and a mediastinal mass. In this marrow trephine there is near complete replacement of normal haemopoiesis by malignant cells—an almost unprecedented occurrence in malignant germ-cell tumours.

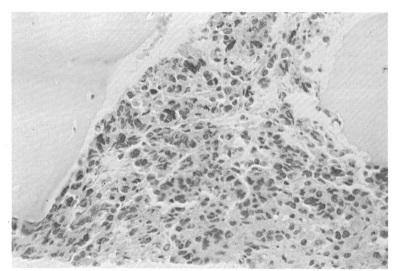

12.31 Malignant germ cell tumour: seminoma with yolk sac elements
Mediastinal mass stained to show alpha-fetoprotein (AFP)

Yolk sac (endodermal sinus) differentiation is demonstrated by the presence of AFP (yellow–brown) in the cells on the right of the picture. Same case as 12.30. This specific 'stain' is important because there is an intriguing and, as yet, unexplained association between malignant germ cell tumours and acute myelo-monocytic (M4) leukaemia.

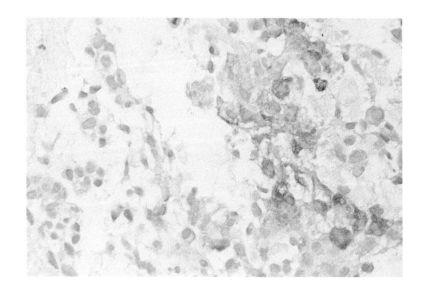

12.32 Ependymoma
Bone-marrow aspirate

Clumps of tumour cells are seen. They have no specific identifying features. This is a rare instance of metastatic ependymoma in a 7-year-old boy who, 2 years before, had a ventriculo-atrial shunt inserted at the time of partial removal of a posterior cranial fossa tumour.

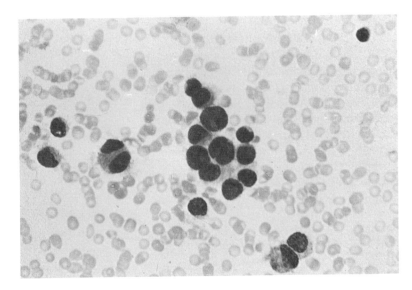

12.33 Ependymoma
Bone marrow trephine; HE

Trephine biopsy from the same patient as in 12.32 showing areas of tumour infiltration and reactive fibrosis alongside some normal haemopoeisis.

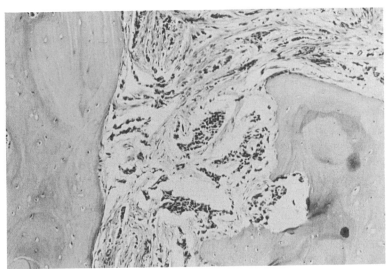

13
Aplastic anaemia

13.1 Fanconi's anaemia
Bone marrow trephine biopsy; HE

This disorder is a constitutional aplastic anaemia: constitutional disorders associated with marrow hypoplasia include dyskeratosis congenita and familial aplasia without congenital anomalies (Estren and Dameshek).

In Fanconi's anaemia the congenital anomalies are usually noted by early infancy but haematological changes are rarely evident before 18 months and can be delayed until the second decade. Thrombocytopenia often precedes the development of pancytopenia. In this 12-year-old boy, marrow hypoplasia had become severe. As with other conditions displaying chromosome breakages, there is a strong association with development of leukaemia. This child died of acute myeloid leukaemia. See 2.64 and 2.65 for dyserythropoietic changes in this disorder.

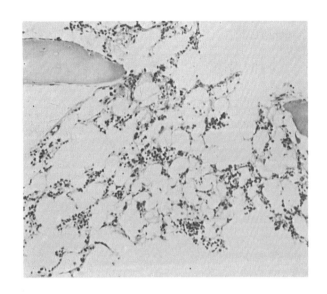

13.2 Idiopathic acquired aplastic anaemia
Bone marrow trephine biopsy; HE

Most cases of aplastic anaemia in childhood are acquired and no cause is found. The marrow biopsy shows the patchy but markedly reduced cellularity and increased fat spaces typical of this disorder.

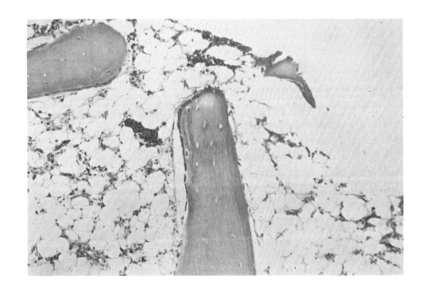

13.3   Moderate acquired aplastic anaemia
Bone marrow trephine biopsy; HE

Most cases of aplastic anaemia in childhood are acquired and no cause is found. The trephine in this cause shows reduced cellularity with occasional clusters of marrow cells. The patient had moderate aplastic anaemia with Hb 8.9 g/dl, platelets $74 \times 10^9/l$, and WBC $1.1 \times 10^9/l$.

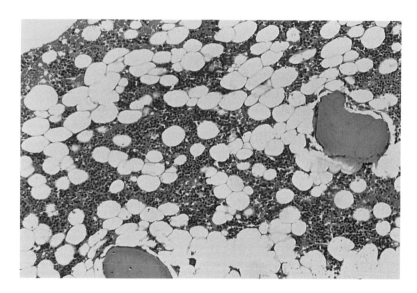

13.4   Severe acquired aplastic anaemia
Bone marrow trephine biopsy; HE

Although the cellularity can be patchy, the trephine in this case was almost entirely devoid of cells.

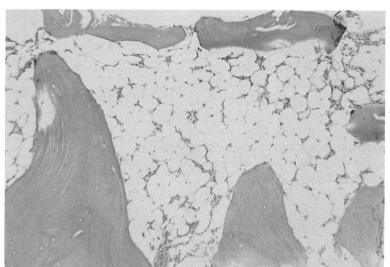

13.5   Aplastic anaemia
Blood film; Kleihauer stain

Hb F-containing red cells are demonstrated because of their resistance to acid elution. In some patients with aplastic anaemia the Hb F is raised, occasionally as high as 15 per cent. This plate shows an increased percentage of cells in a heterogeneous distribution. Some 'ghost' cells contain little or no Hb F.

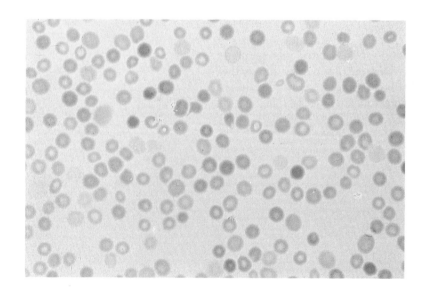

13.6 Post-hepatitis marrow aplasia
Bone marrow

Aplastic anaemia following hepatitis A carries a poor prognosis. A bone marrow particle with greatly decreased cellularity is shown.

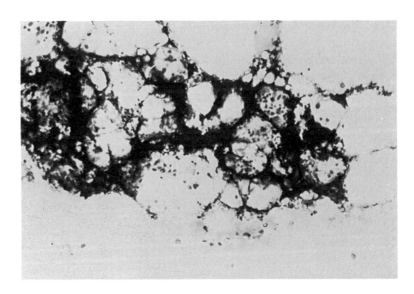

13.7 Post-cytotoxic chemotherapy aplasia
Bone marrow trephine biopsy; HE

The cellularity is grossly decreased following a course of intensive chemotherapy in a patient with RAEB. Similar appearances may be seen following ablative chemo-radiotherapy as conditioning for bone marrow transplantation.

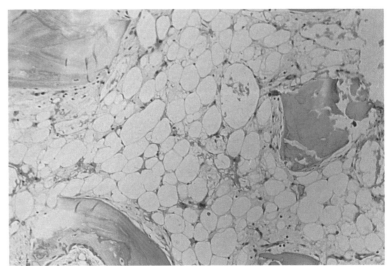

13.8 Hereditary spherocytosis—parvovirus-induced aplasia
Blood film

A 7-year-old boy with hereditary spherocytosis presented with an 'aplastic crisis' (Hb 4.5 g/dl and reticulocytopenia). IgM to parvovirus B19 was demonstrated.

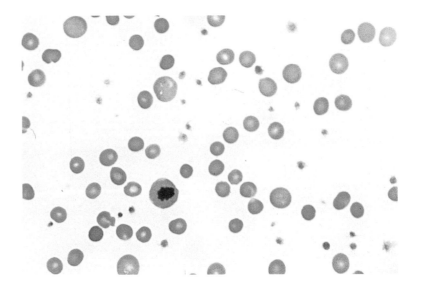

13.9   Parvovirus-induced aplasia
Bone marrow

Parvovirus can cause aplasia of other marrow elements although it usually produces severe anaemia. It has recently been recognized that bizarre giant cells are often present in the marrow in these cases. Sometimes these present as bare nuclei and in other cases resemble early pronormoblasts. They always have very prominent nucleoli.

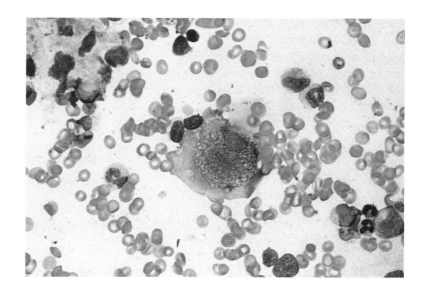

13.10   Parvovirus-induced aplasia
Bone marrow; see 13.8

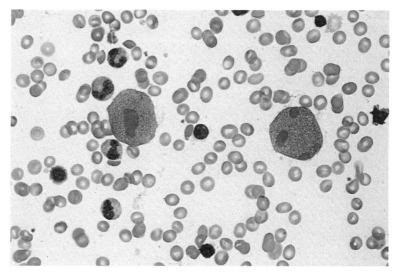

14
Neonatal and perinatal disorders

14.1 Fetal blood
Blood

Blood taken from a 23-week fetus. The
red cells are larger than in later life (MCV
≥ 105 fl). A single nucleated red cell is
seen.

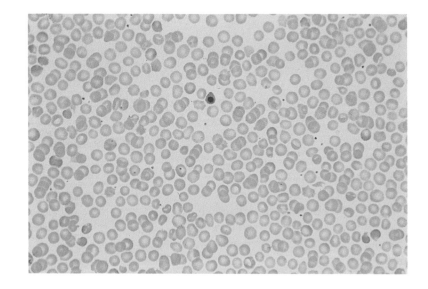

14.2 Cord blood
Blood

Sample from a healthy normal-term baby.
There is anisocytosis with macrocytes and
a few circulating nucleated red cells.
Irregularly contracted cells are also
common. The MCV is still high compared
with adults (MCV ≥ 100fl)—see Chapter
18.

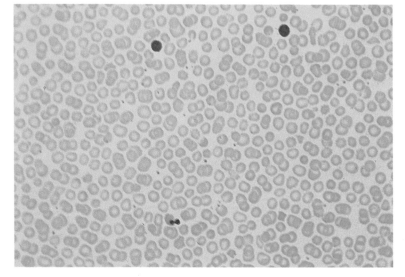

14.3 Neonatal marrow
Bone marrow

There are fewer erythroblasts and more lymphocytes in neonatal marrows compared with those of older children.

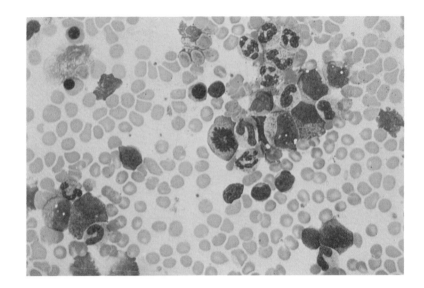

14.4 Neonatal marrow
Bone marrow

An abundance of iron from the post-natal red cell 'cull' is to be found in neonatal marrows and iron laden macrophages are not uncommon.

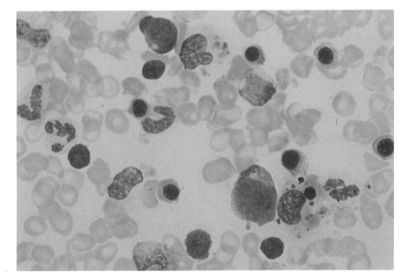

14.5 Neonatal marrow
Bone marrow

A Perls' stain for iron confirms the iron loading of macrophages described above.

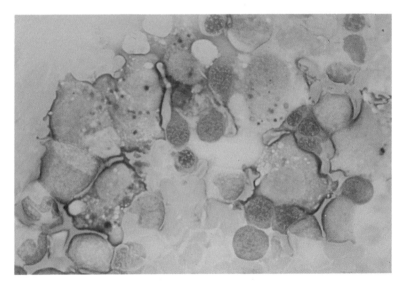

14.6 The 'stressed' neonate—respiratory distress syndrome (RDS)
Blood

Poikilocytosis and irregularly contracted cells are common features of blood films from sick neonates, sometimes giving rise to the nebulous diagnosis of 'infantile pyknocytosis', an ill-defined entity best ignored. Premature infant of 27 weeks on day 3.

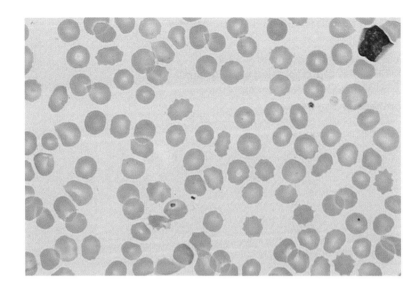

14.7 The 'stressed' neonate—respiratory distress syndrome
Blood

Nucleated red cells and Howell–Jolly bodies indicate functional hyposplenism. Same patient as 14.6.

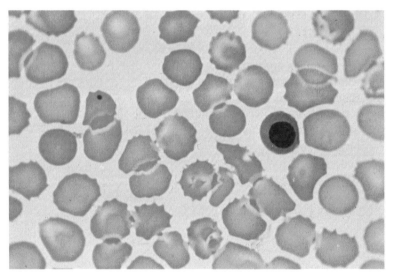

14.8 The 'stressed' neonate—respiratory distress syndrome
Blood

RDS is an occasional cause of consumption coagulopathy (disseminated intravascular coagulation) as in this case where red cell fragmentation/damage is associated with profound thrombocytopenia.

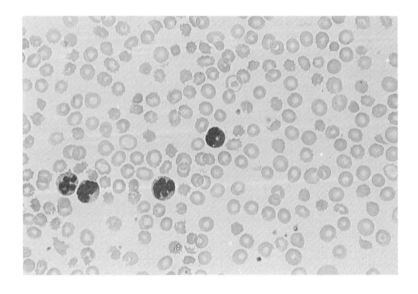

14.9   The 'stressed' neonate—sepsis
Blood

One-day-old term neonate with a
septicaemia. Note spherocytes and band-
form neutrophil. Neutropenia often
complicates this picture.

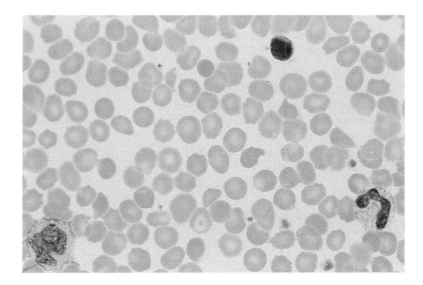

14.10   The 'stressed' neonate—sepsis
Blood

Vacuolation of mononuclear cells is seen
in septic neonates and very occasionally
intracellular microbes are visible as in this
case. The organisms are coagulase-
negative staphylococci from an infant
with an umbilical catheter *in situ*.

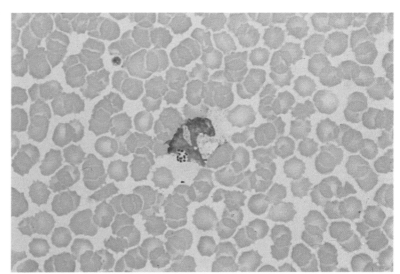

14.11   The 'stressed' neonate—sepsis
Blood

Disseminated intravascular coagulation
commonly complicates neonatal
septicaemia (from any cause) as well as
the respiratory distress syndrome (see 14.7
above). If the condition persists for more
than 24–48 hours, fragmented red cells as
shown will appear in association with
profound thrombocytopenia.

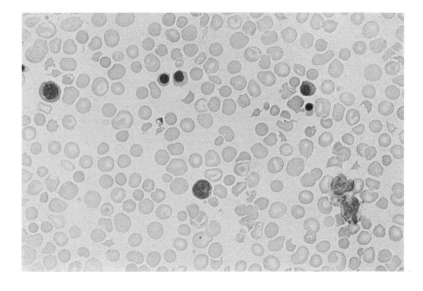

14.12 The 'stressed' neonate—sepsis
Blood

Twelve-day-old neonate with a tracheo-oesophageal fistula and pneumonia. Pyknocytosis, polychromasia, and anisocytosis. Similar red-cell abnormalities can be produced by a variety of different pathological conditions.

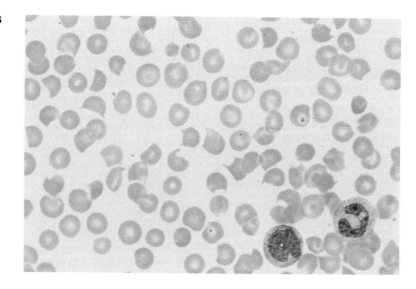

14.13 Haemolytic disease of the newborn—feto:maternal haemorrhage
Kleihauer film of maternal blood

Shows a massive transplacental haemorrhage with 20 000 fetal cells per 50 low-power fields.

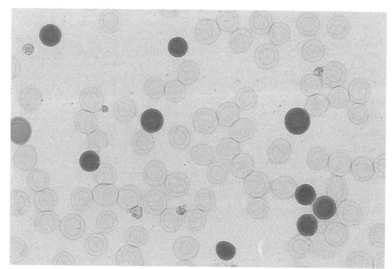

14.14 Haemolytic disease of the newborn—feto:maternal haemorrhage
Blood (maternal)

Shows macrocyte of probable fetal origin. The baby was born anaemic (7 g/dl) with no evidence of haemolysis.

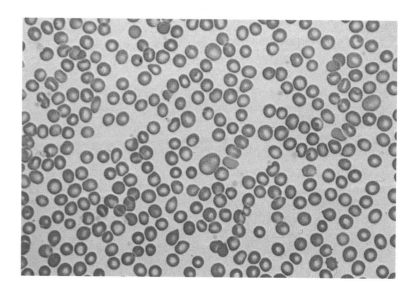

14.15 Haemolytic disease of the newborn—isoimmune due to anti-D
Blood (cord blood)

Numerous erythroblasts and polychromatic macrocytes; occasional spherocytes; anaemia. The direct antiglobulin test is strongly positive, and the baby's cells are coated with maternal anti-D.

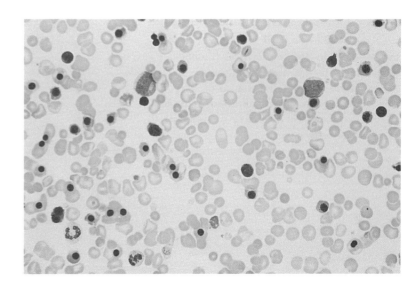

14.16 Haemolytic disease of the newborn—ABO haemolytic disease
Blood

Usually less severe than Rhesus haemolytic disease, with a negative or only weakly positive direct antiglobulin test. ABO disease presents 24–72 hours after birth with jaundice being more clinically striking than anaemia. Spherocytes are a feature rather than an occasional finding. The problem usually arises with group A babies being born to group O mothers.

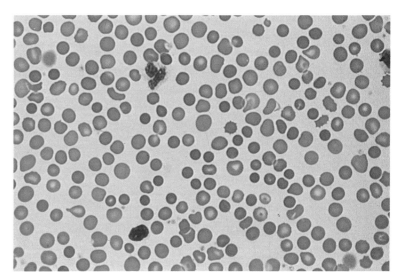

14.17 'TORCH' infection—cytomegalovirus
Bone marrow

All the congenital 'TORCH' infections (toxoplasmosis, rubella, cytomegalovirus, and herpes simplex) together with congenital syphilis can produce a similar haematological picture in the neonate, with hepatosplenomegaly, jaundice, anaemia and thrombocytopenia. The marrow (as in this case) may contain cells morphologically similar to lymphoblasts. This baby was born with purpura and hepatosplenomegaly. Confusion with congenital leukaemia can arise (see below).

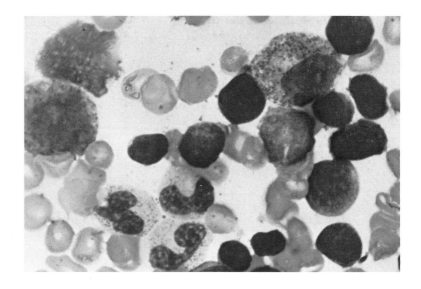

14.18 'TORCH' infection—cytomegalovirus
Bone marrow
Further material from the same patient as 14.17.

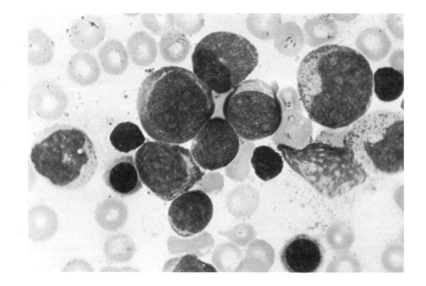

14.19 'TORCH' infection—cytomegalovirus
Bone marrow
Same patient as 14.17.

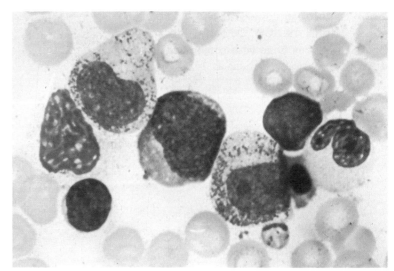

14.20 Reticular dysgenesis
Bone marrow
This child suffered recurrent infections starting in the neonatal period. At the age of 9 months he was shown to have neutropenia, lymphopenia, and absent serum immunoglobulins. Reticular dysgenesis, a very rare form of severe combined immune deficiency, was diagnosed. The bone marrow shows depletion of lymphoid and granulocyte precursors, particularly mature forms. The baby was successfully treated by allogeneic bone marrow transplantation.

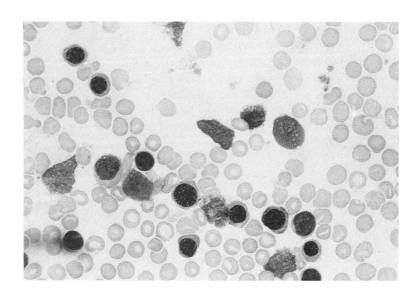

14.21   Infantile osteopetrosis
Blood

Gross leucoerythroblastosis can occasionally be confused with leukaemia. The patient was a 6-month-old boy with pallor since birth and massive splenomegaly. The condition is an inherited functional deficiency of osteoclasts.

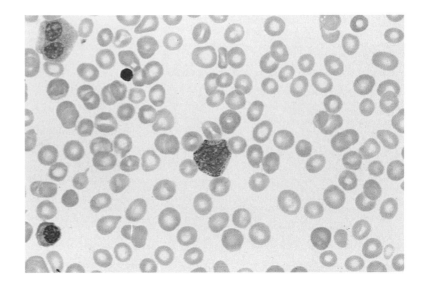

14.22   Infantile osteopetrosis
Bone marrow trephine

Dense cancellous bone with constricted marrow space. Same patient as 14.21.

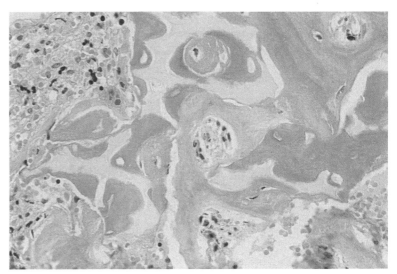

14.23   Infantile osteopetrosis
Bone marrow trephine

The trephine appearances vary from patient to patient but there is invariably a gross excess of cancellous bone. Another child with the same condition.

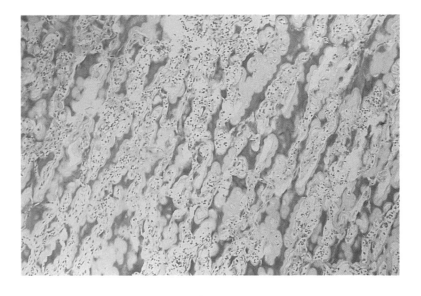

14.24 Neonatal sideroblastic anaemia
Blood

An anaemic neonate with gross anisochromia and anisocytosis coupled with a dual population of red cells due to congenital sideroblastic anaemia. This gross disorder of heme synthesis may be caused by a defect of mitochondrial DNA (Pearson's syndrome). (See also Chapter 2.)

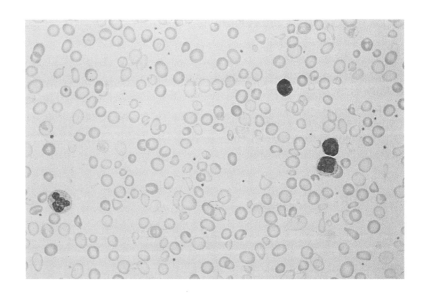

14.25 Neonatal sideroblastic anaemia
Bone marrow

Marrow erythroblasts from the patient illustrated in 14.24 stained with Perls' stain for iron and showing the characteristic 'ring' appearance with a collar of siderotic granules around the nucleus.

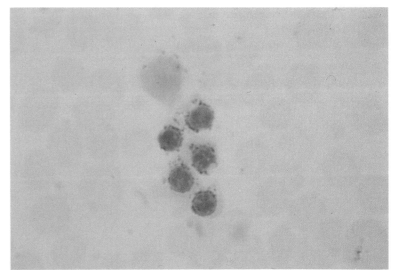

14.26 Neonatal haemolytic uraemic syndrome (HUS)
Blood

Rarely, HUS can be seen in neonates. It is not usually the epidemic form associated with enterotoxins from Gram-negative bacteria, and carries a worse outlook. There is red cell fragmentation and thrombocytopenia without other evidence of consumption coagulopathy.

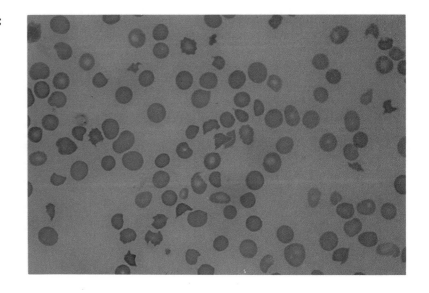

14.27   Congenital leukaemia (monocytic)
Bone marrow

Congenital leukaemia is very rare, and usually monocyte-related. The morphology is similar to that seen in acquired M5 AML (see Chapter 8). Discoid skin lesions due to cutaneous infiltration are often present.

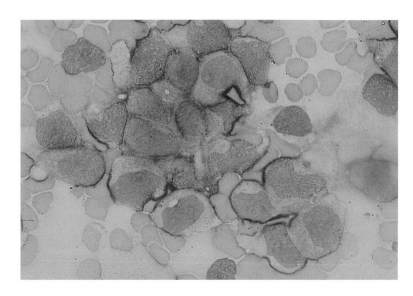

14.28   Congenital leukaemia (monocytic)
Bone marrow; esterase stain

The monocyte lineage can be demonstrated by positive staining with α-naphthyl acetate esterase.

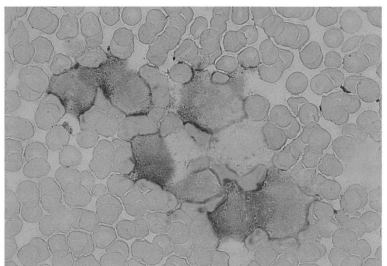

14.29   Congenital leukaemia (lymphoblastic)
Blood

Even less commonly, other types of leukaemia can present at birth, and this is an acute lymphoblastic example. It did not have the immunological or cytogenetic features of 'common' childhood ALL. Such children seldom fare well.

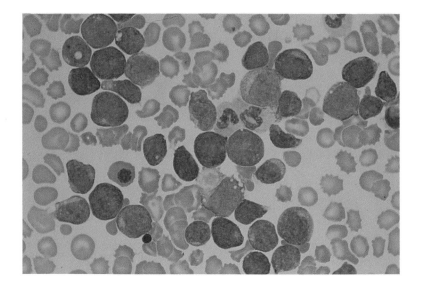

**14.30 Congenital leukaemia
(lymphoblastic)**
Bone marrow
The marrow from the patient illustrated in
14.29.

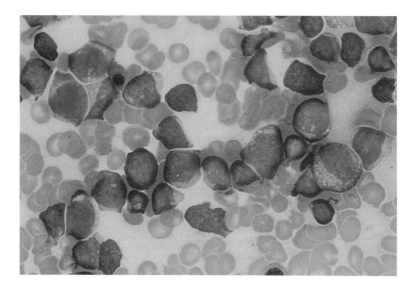

15
Parasites and opportunistic infections

15.1 Malaria; *Plasmodium vivax*, early trophozoites (signet forms)
Blood film

This plate shows two cells infected with trophozoites. One contains three distinct signet forms—a single parasite is much more usual. Schuffner's dots are not present at this early stage.

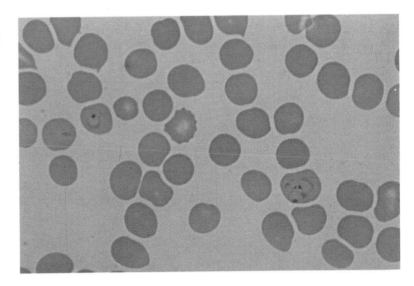

15.2 Malaria; *Plasmodium vivax*, developing trophozoite
Blood film

The red cell at the centre contains a single trophozoite and pink–red stippling (Schuffner's dots) which is difficult to see, and is not in every infected cell. Schuffner's dots are not seen in *P. malariae*.

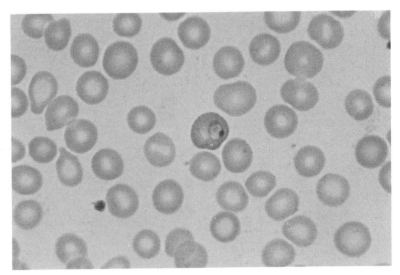

15.3 Malaria; *Plasmodium vivax*, developing trophozoites
Blood film

The parasite shows a coarse irregular (amoeboid) shape of chromatin which appears as dots or threads. Scattered fine brown pigment granules are present. The pigment increases with development. In *P. falciparum* there are few pigment granules observed at any stage.

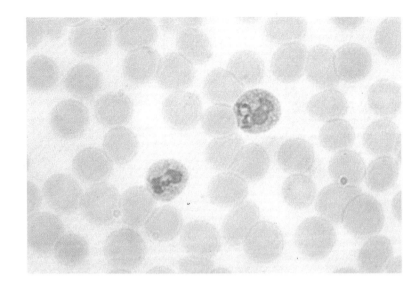

15.4 Malaria; *Plasmodium vivax*, schizonts
Blood film

The non-segmented schizonts represent a phase of the asexual cycle later than the trophozoite. At this stage Schuffner's dots may be numerous around the periphery of the infected red cell.

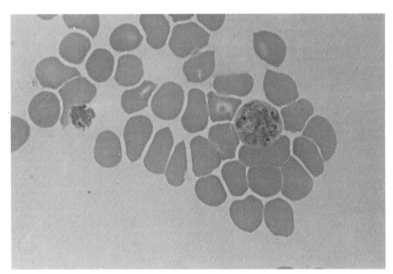

15.5 Malaria; *Plasmodium vivax*, schizonts
Blood film

Gradual condensation of the chromatin occurs prior to the final development of the merozoites.

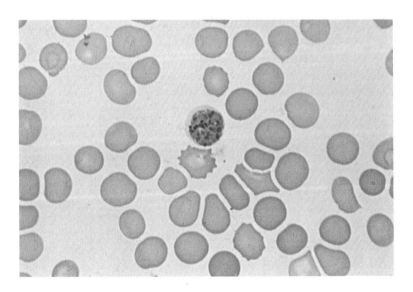

15.6 Malaria; *Plasmodium vivax*, schizogony
Blood film

The plate shows a segmented schizont just prior to separation of individual merozoites. Typically there are 16 merozoites, but the number can be 12–18. In *P. malariae*, 8 is usual (6–12).

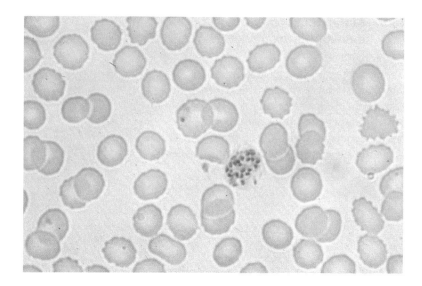

15.7 Malaria; *Plasmodium vivax*, microgametocytes
Blood film

The microgametocytes may be numerous in the blood film. They fill the enlarged red cell and contain numerous pigment granules. Schuffner's dots are not present at this stage.

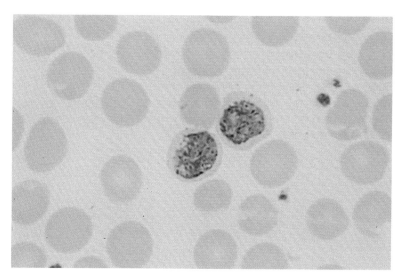

15.8 Malaria; *Plasmodium vivax*, exflagellation (microgametes)
Blood film

A developing trophozoite, complete with Schuffner's dots, is shown together with an exflagellated microgamete.

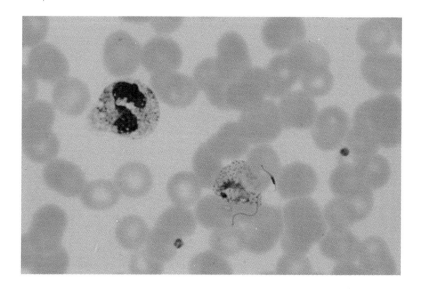

15.9   Malaria; *Plasmodium vivax*, exflagellation (microgamete) Blood film

A free microgamete is present with a distinct central chromatin spot. This serves to help distinguish this form from *Trypanosoma* where the nucleus and undulating membrane are at one end (see 15.23).

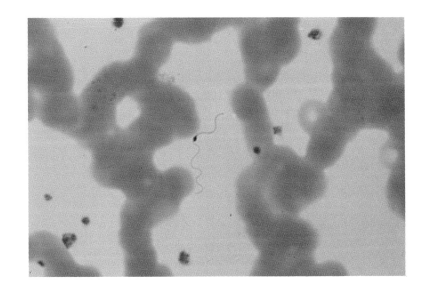

15.10   Malaria; *Plasmodium vivax* Bone marrow film

Occasional ring trophozoite forms were found in the marrow from this patient who presented with hepatosplenomegaly and fever. No parasites were initially detected in the peripheral blood.

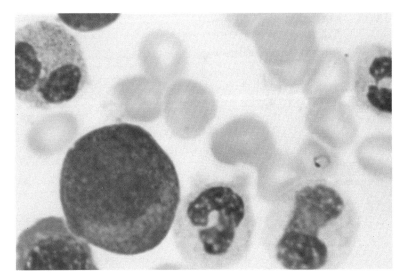

15.11   Malaria; *Plasmodium falciparum*, ring trophozoite Blood film

The ring form of *P. falciparum* is smaller and more delicate than that of *P. vivax*. Multiple infected cells are common. Maurer's clefts (reddish clefts or blotches), common in the developing trophozoite, are not shown here. Few pigment granules are observed in *P. vivax* in contrast to other forms of malaria.

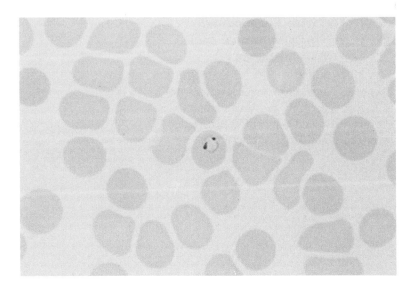

15.12 Malaria; *Plasmodium falciparum*
Blood film

Segmented mature schizonts (containing 6–12 merozoites) are present in this illustration (lower right) together with a signet form (upper left).

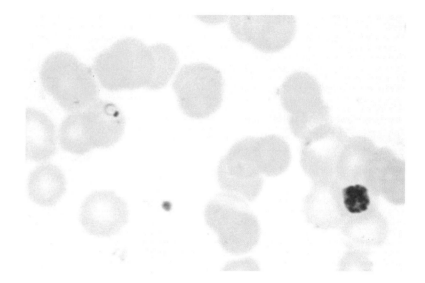

15.13 Malaria; *Plasmodium falciparum*
'Thick' blood film

The thick film, in skilled hands, is quick to make and is the best preparation for general clinical use. By this method all red cells are lysed and the diagnostic chromatin dots consequently stand out. Here the heavily stained cells are white blood cells on a background of *P. falciparum* chromatin.

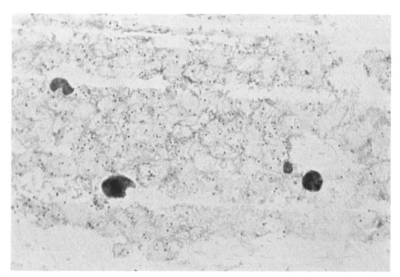

15.14 Malaria; *Plasmodium falciparum*, sexual cycle, microgametocyte
Blood film

The male gametocyte (microgametocyte) is shown. The pink and blue cytoplasm is characteristic and pigment is distributed throughout the large nucleus.

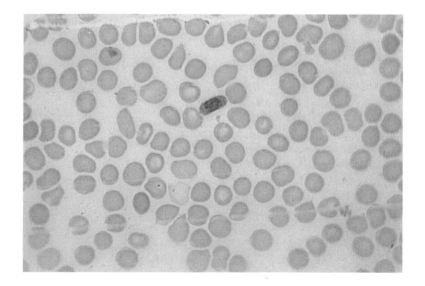

15.15 Malaria; *Plasmodium falciparum*, sexual cycle, macrogametocyte
Blood film

The female gametocyte (macrogametocyte) with its sharply rounded or pointed ends and dense small nucleus is illustrated here. The cytoplasm is typically deeper blue than that of the microgametocyte.

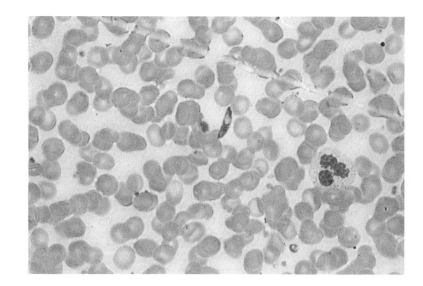

15.16 Malaria; *Plasmodium ovale*
Blood film

Developing trophozoite. This occupies up to one-third of the red cell, which becomes irregular and pointed. Schuffner's dots are present and are usually more prominent than in *P. vivax*.

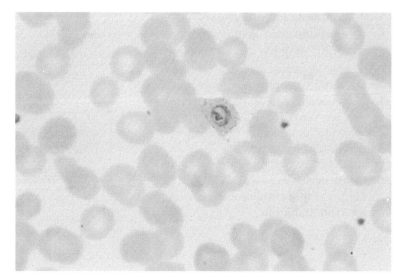

15.17 Malaria; *Plasmodium malariae*
Blood film

The schizonts are very similar to those of *P. ovale*. Merozoites typically are 6–12, with 8 being usual. In the trophozoite stage Schuffner's dots are not present.

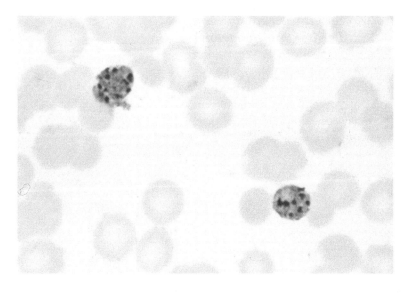

15.18 Malaria; *Plasmodium malariae*
Blood film

The macrogametocyte is similar to that of *P. vivax*.

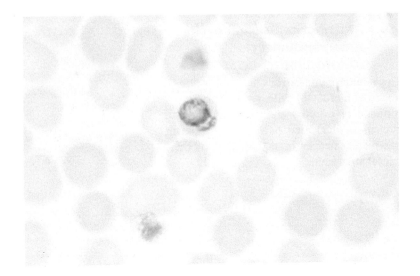

15.19 Visceral leishmaniasis (*Leishmania donovani*)
Bone marrow

The 3-year-old patient had just returned, with fever and hepatosplenomegaly, to the UK after a holiday in Jordan. Here the parasites have invaded a macrophage. Each parasite (amastigote, Leishman–Donovan body) has a dense trophonucleus and a less densely staining kinetoplast, which are also readily visible in histological preparations stained with haematoxylin and eosin.

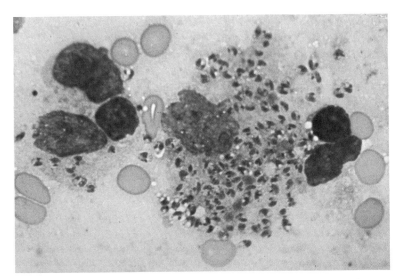

15.20 Visceral leishmaniasis, (*Leishmania donovani*)
Bone marrow

This infant had returned from a holiday in Malta, and became unwell with pancytopenia and hepatosplenomegaly. The amastigotes are present in the cytoplasm of a mononuclear cell.

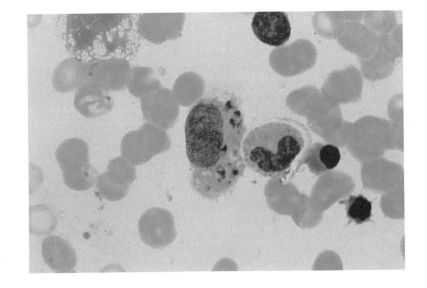

15.21 Visceral leishmaniasis, (*Leishmania donovani*) Bone marrow

From the same patient as in 15.20. Here the amastigotes are lying free.

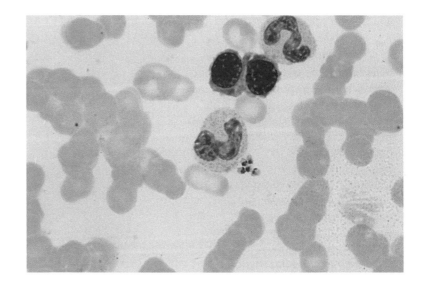

15.22 *Trypanosoma brucei rhodesiense* (Rhodesian sleeping sickness) Blood film

These parasites are transmitted by the tsetse fly. This patient had been on a hunting expedition to the Zambesi valley and presented with an encephalitic illness. The plate shows the trypomastiogote's undulating membrane, flagellum, nucleus, and kinetoplast.

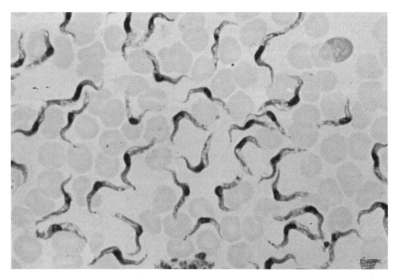

15.23 *Trypanosoma brucei rhodesiense* (Rhodesian sleeping sickness) Blood film

The appearances are indistinguishable from *T. gambiense*, but the chronic nature of *T. brucei gambiense* infection helps to differentiate it from the more acute effects of *T. brucei rhodesiense*.

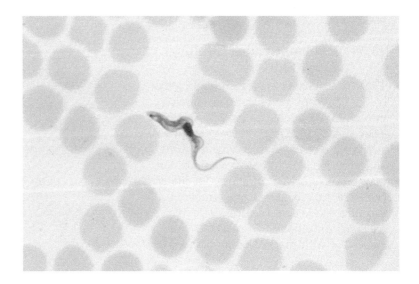

15.24 *Trypanosoma cruzi* (Chagas' disease)
Blood film

This parasite is indigenous to South America. The trypomastigote has a very large terminal kinetoplast, a large nucleus, and is typically C-shaped in stained preparations. The clinical presentation in children is usually remitting fever, muscle pain, lymphadenopathy, oedema, and lesions of the skin (chagomas), or of conjunctiva (Romana's sign). Myocarditis, encephalitis, and progressive intestinal dysfunction also occur. *T. cruzi* metamorphose in tissue macrophages and have leishmanial (amastigote) forms which are indistinguishable from *L. donovani.*

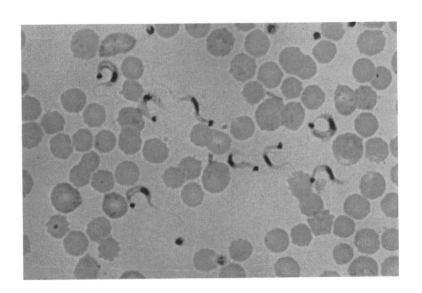

15.25 Microfilariasis, *Wuchereria bancrofti*
Blood film

Filariae are members of the Nematoda. Their larval forms—microfilariae—are found in the blood, especially at night. Chronic consequences of filarial infection include lymphangitis and elephantiasis (rare in children). *Wuchereria bancrofti* is sheathed and the nuclei do not extend to the tip of the tail. *Brugia malayi* is similar in its habit and form; its nuclei extend to the tail. Other microfilariae may be found in the blood (e.g *Dipetalonema perstans, Dipetalonema streptocerca,* and *Mansonella ozzardi*) but these are unsheathed and seem to be non-pathogenic.

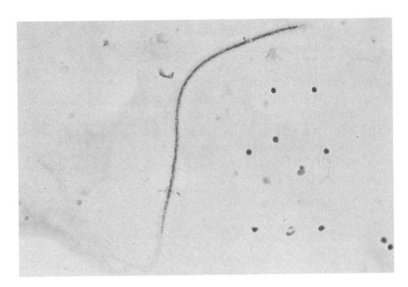

15.26 Loa-loa (Calabar swelling)
Blood film

These microfiliarae are transmitted by flies of the Chrysops genus and will develop into adult worms up to 7 cm in length. They cause soft tissue swellings (fugitive swellings) especially on the hands, arms, and periorbitally. Although the infection may be chronic, the prognosis for life is excellent. Loa-loa are demonstrable in a day-time blood film in contrast to *W. bancrofti.* Infection is frequently associated with marked eosinophilia.

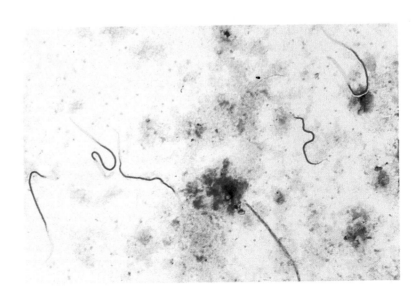

15.27 Loa-loa
Blood film

The microfilariae are sheathed and measure up to 300 μm long. The nuclei extend to the tip of the tail. They appear more kinked and bent than *W. bancrofti*.

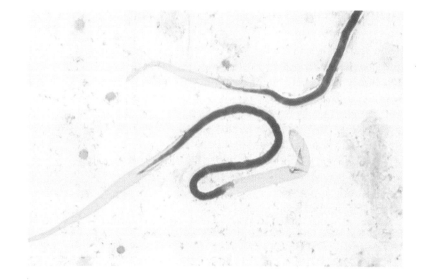

15.28 Babesia
Blood film

Babesiosis is a tick-borne disease with mild symptoms of fever, malaise, muscle pain, and haemolytic anaemia. The organisms are present in red blood cells and have a variety of appearances. Here the coccoid form is seen.

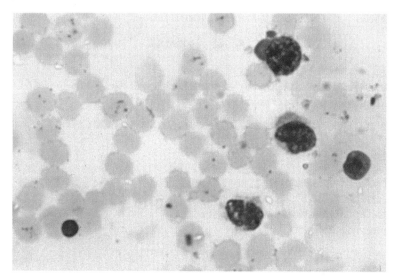

15.29 Babesia
Blood film

The organism also has some resemblance to the ring trophozoite form of *P. falciparum*.

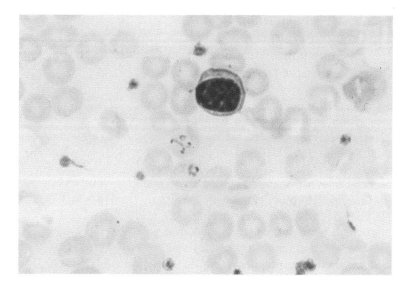

15.30   Borrelia
Blood film

Lyme disease is caused by the tick-borne spirochaete *Borrelia burgdorferi* and infection gives rise to malaise, fatigue, arthralgia, myalgia, and fever. It is considered to be a progressive multisystem disease. The first sign is a migrating annular skin lesion developing at the site of the tick bite. Other forms, particularly *Borrelia recurrentis* transmitted by the human body louse, give rise to relapsing fever. The spirochaetes circulate and multiply in body fluids and do not enter cells.

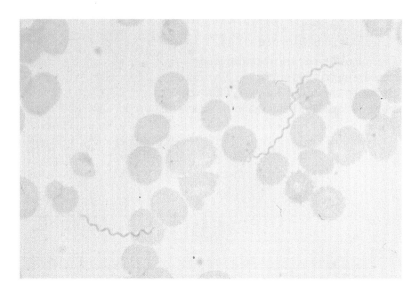

15.31   *Candida albicans* (Moniliasis)
Bone marrow trephine; H and E

This teenage patient had had a bone marrow transplant for leukaemia 3 months previously. Haemopoietic reconstitution had occurred but the patient developed persistent fever. *C. albicans* was cultured from both blood and bone marrow. The fungus (mainly hyphal forms) is readily seen in this section. A PAS reaction or silver methanamine would show the fungus more clearly.

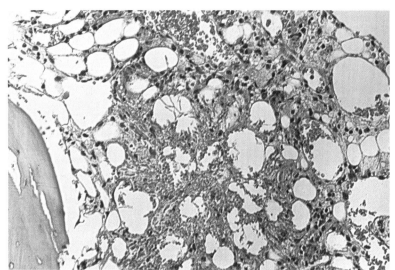

15.32   *Mycobacterium avium intracellulare*
Bone marrow section; H and E

Large macrophages fill and have replaced the bone marrow of this patient. Their cytoplasm containing the organism has a grey granular appearance. This patient, a 12-year-old boy presented with a 10-month history of PUO and a tippable spleen, and on the basis of investigations was considered to have generalized polyarteritis. He was treated with steroids. He later had vomiting, diarrhoea, abdominal pain, and epistaxis, and died. He had been immunocompromised and had succumbed to this opportunistic infection, which is also found in other immunosuppressed patients (e.g. HIV infection, leukaemic, and other patients with bone marrow transplants).

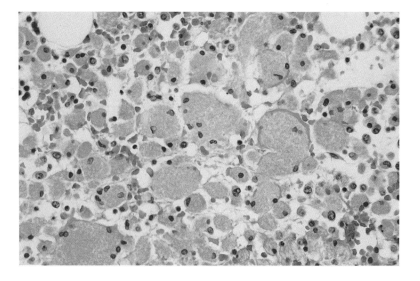

15.33 *Mycobacterium avium intracellulare*

Bone marrow section; Ziehl–Neelsen

The large macrophages in the marrow are filled with red-staining mycobacteria. This section is from the same case as shown in 15.32.

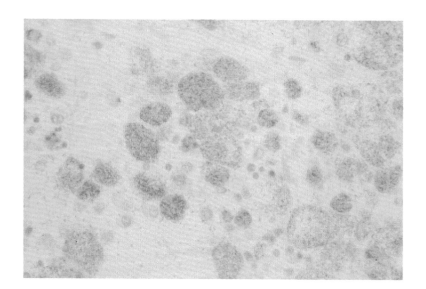

16
Storage disorders

Visceral storage disorders are recognized by the presence of foamy cells in bone marrow aspirates. Not all foamy cells are storage cells. Occasional foamy cells, or isolated foamy cells, are not usually an indication of a storage disorder, and only when they occur in large numbers should a storage disorder be considered. Their morphology and staining characteristics with a limited range of histochemical tests, should be interpreted in conjunction with a full clinical history. Many of the lysosomal storage disorders show vacuolation of peripheral lymphocytes, and these changes also need careful interpretation in the light of the clinical presentation.

16.1 Normal marrow
Bone marrow
Not all foamy cells are storage cells. This cell is a normal fat cell and occurs in normal marrow in small numbers. The vacuoles are less well defined than those of most storage cells.

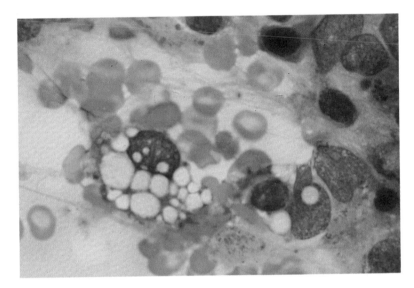

16.2 Blood film, not storage disease
Small vacuoles, usually single, may be found in activated lymphocytes. This is not an indication of a storage disease. Similarly, monocytes which are vacuolated are a normal phenomenon in anticoagulated blood samples.

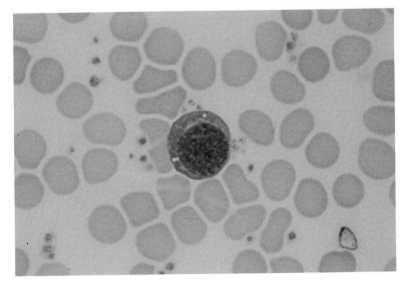

Gaucher's disease

The **infantile** form presents in infancy with marked hepatosplenomegaly, failure to thrive, and psychomotor retardation. The **juvenile** form presents around 3–4 years with hepatosplenomegaly and myoclonic fits. Mental retardation and a defect in horizontal gaze (in contrast to the vertical gaze palsy of Niemann–Pick disease type C) often also develop. The **adult** form presents from 2–3 years onwards. Bone pain and thrombocytopenia are common in long-standing cases. The activity of β-glucocerebrosidase is deficient. Vacuolation of lymphocytes is not found.

16.3 Gaucher's disease
Bone marrow

The typical Gaucher cell has a striped appearance often likened to crumpled tissue paper. However, this appearance is not always as clear as in the illustration and cells may appear more vacuolated. The Gaucher cells are sometimes multinucleate and are PAS-positive. Similar cells, but with a more striking blue cytoplasmic striped appearance, occur in G_{M1}-gangliosidosis type II (see 16.23). Foamy cells and pseudo-Gaucher cells may occur in 'adult' type chronic granulocytic leukaemia (see 9.26) and in other conditions of overload of the macrophage system.

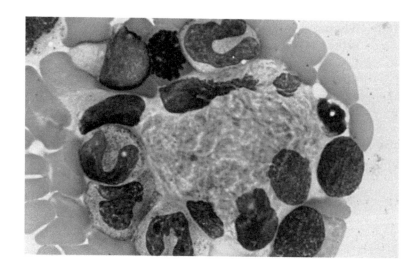

16.4 Gaucher's disease
Bone marrow; acid phosphatase (Gömöri) reaction

More storage cells are found in the infantile form, and are readily revealed by their acid phosphatase activity (tartrate-stable). Megakaryocytes have only fine granular activity in a portion of the cell. The acid phosphatase reaction will identify all storage cells and macrophages in a marrow film.

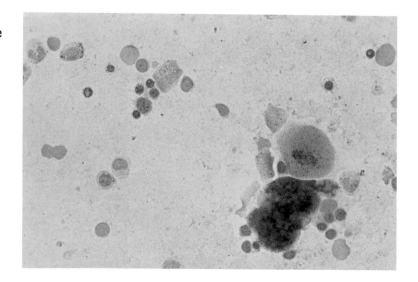

Niemann–Pick disease

Classification: The classification of Niemann–Pick disease is now based on the enzymatic characteristics of the individual disorders. Types A (acute infantile, neuropathic) and B (chronic, non-neuropathic juvenile and adult) are both deficient in lysosomal sphingomyelinase activity. Type C (acute infantile, juvenile, and adult forms exist) has normal sphingomyelinase activity but cultured fibroblasts exhibit deficient cholesterol esterification. Type D, formerly the Nova Scotian variant, is now regarded as type C having the same biochemical and morphological characteristics. Type E, formerly the adult type, is classed as type B. Vacuolated lymphocytes, similar to those in 16.12, are found in peripheral blood films in type A only.

16.5   Niemann-Pick disease (type A, infantile)
Bone marrow

Foamy storage cells, generally with uniformly sized vacuoles in any one cell, are prominent throughout the cell. Only rarely is an engulfed red cell or some nuclear debris present. Vacuolated lymphocytes can also be found in the marrow film.

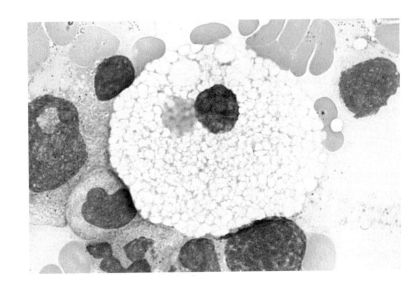

16.6   Niemann–Pick disease (type A, infantile)
Bone marrow; Sudan black for lipid

The Niemann–Pick cells stain weakly with Sudan black, but will show red birefringence in polarized light after this stain. Unstained cells also exhibit birefringence in contrast to those of Niemann–Pick disease type C.

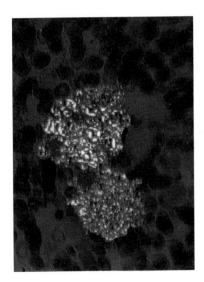

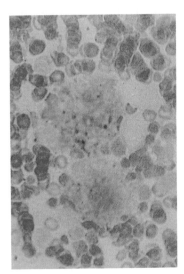

16.7 Niemann–Pick disease (type B, adult)
Bone marrow

Abundant 'sea-blue' histiocytes are present and these are often so prominent that the smaller population of foamy cells may be overlooked. The 'sea-blue' cells are packed with blue-staining granules which are also PAS-Positive, sudanophilic, and brightly autofluorescent indicating their lipofuscin content. Cells with lesser numbers of granules should not be called 'sea-blue'. Occasional 'sea-blue' histiocytes are found in the juvenile patients, and also in Niemann–Pick disease type C (see 16.11) and Fabry's disease.

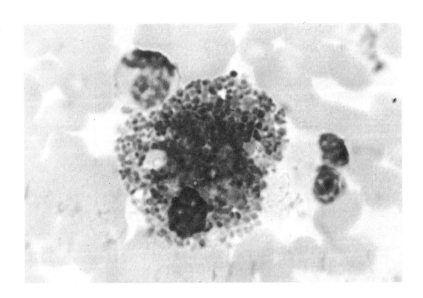

16.8 Niemann–Pick disease type C
Bone marrow from an infant

The numerous cells resemble the classic Niemann–Pick cell, but differ in having vacuoles of varying sizes in the same cell. The vacuoles are also less well defined. Densely staining nuclear debris (normoblast probably although other nuclear forms are also seen) is a common finding within the cells. The infantile form usually (around 60 per cent of patients) presents with neonatal hepatitis and significant splenomegaly. Bone marrow aspiration, rather than a liver biopsy, is the investigation of choice in this circumstance.

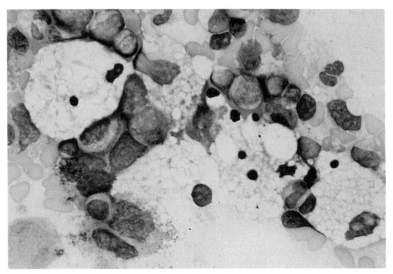

16.9 Niemann–Pick disease type C
Bone marrow

In the older child presenting, often with isolated splenomegaly only, the nuclear debris is more prominent than seen in the infant. No birefringence is found. The cells are strongly PAS-positive. Rare 'sea-blue' histiocytes with characteristics similar to those shown in 16.7 may be found, their numbers increasing with the age of the patient.

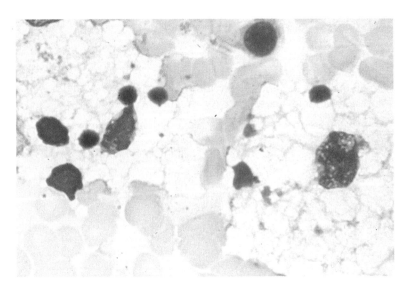

16.10   Niemann–Pick disease type C
   Bone marrow; Sudan black for
   lipid

The storage cells are usually unstained (upper right) but the granules in the 'sea-blue' cells are stained grey-black indicating a lipofuscin-like material rather than neutral fat.

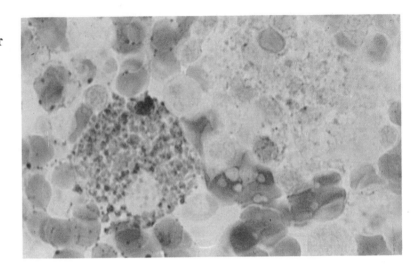

16.11   Niemann–Pick disease type C
   Bone marrow from
   heterozygote

Heterozygotes also show the same storage cells as those in affected cases, but to a lesser extent. The index case was a patient who presented with dementia and minimal splenomegaly in the juvenile period. This film was from the younger clinically normal sibling being screened at the request of the parents.

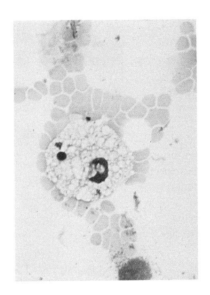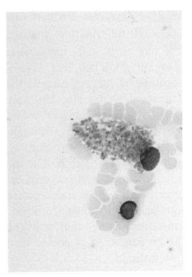

Wolman's disease

The fatal infantile form presents from early infancy with hepatosplenomegaly, failure to thrive, anaemia, and adrenal calcification. The juvenile and adult forms (cholesteryl ester storage disease) in contrast are mild and present with slight hepatosplenomegaly. Lysosomal acid esterase (acid lipase) activity is deficient in each form.

16.12 Wolman's disease (and cholesteryl ester storage disease)
Blood film

Small, well defined cytoplasmic vacuoles up to about six per cell are present in many lymphocytes in Wolman's disease. Fewer cells show this change in cholesteryl ester storage disease. The vacuoles contain neutral fat which can be detected by staining with Oil Red O. Lipaemic serum may make it difficult to decide whether the lipid is intra- or extracellular. Rarely there may be distinct foamy cells in peripheral blood films (see 16.24).

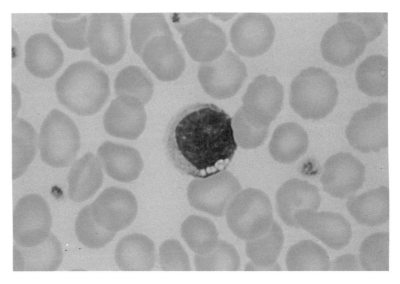

16.13 Wolman's disease (and cholesteryl ester storage disease)
Blood film; acid esterase stain

In the normal patient, acid esterase activity is shown by discrete blocks of reaction product (right-hand picture) in T-lymphocytes. A diffuse strong reaction is found in monocytes. In Wolman's disease and cholesteryl ester storage disease, the reaction in lymphocytes is much weaker or indeed absent (left-hand picture) in most.

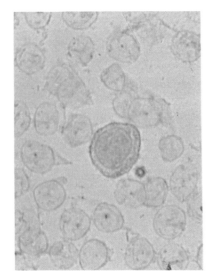
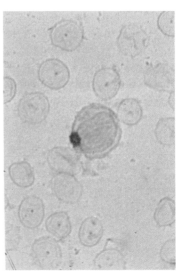

16.14 Wolman's disease
Bone marrow

Large foamy storage cells are present, and are similar to those found in G_{M1}-gangliosidosis type I (see 16.21).

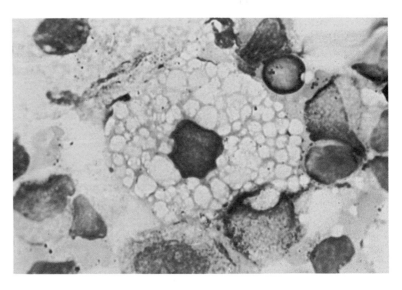

16.15   Wolman's disease
Bone marrow; Oil Red O for neutral fat

The large foamy storage cells are filled with sudanophilic lipid. This is in contrast with all other storage disorders which have only weak or negative reactions for fat. Birefringence (often as maltese cross) is due to the cholesteryl esters and triglycerides. Crystals may develop with storage.

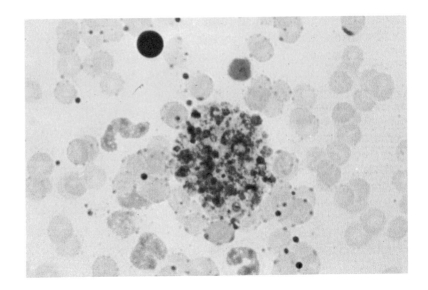

16.16   Wolman's disease
Bone marrow; Nile blue (Cain's method)

The storage cells stain a deep purple/blue due to the presence of free fatty acids as well as the lipid esters.

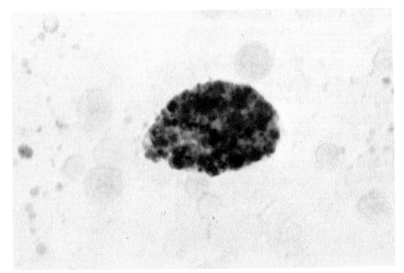

16.17   Cholesteryl ester storage disease
Bone marrow

Fewer storage cells are evident, and their appearance is not as distinctive as those in Wolman's disease.

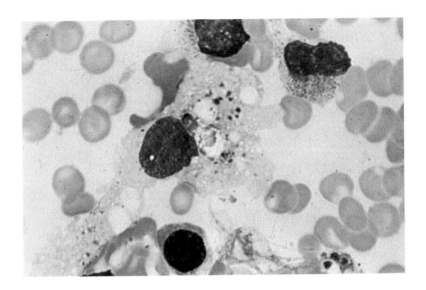

16.18   Cholesteryl ester storage disease
Bone marrow; Oil Red O for neutral lipids

The rare storage cells accumulate neutral fat.

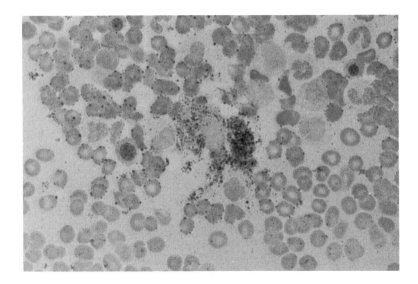

Pompe's disease, juvenile and adult acid maltase deficency

The infantile form (Pompe's disease) presents in early infancy with cardiomegaly, hepato-splenomegaly, and hypotonia. The rarer juvenile and adult forms present with muscle weakness. The activity of acid maltase is deficient in all forms. The simplest test to screen for this group of disorders is to examine blood films for lymphocytic vacuolation and deposition of glycogen within the vacuoles. It is particularly useful in the infant in whom the diagnosis of Pompe's needs to be excluded.

16.19   Pompe's disease (glycogen storage disease type II)
Blood film; PAS after celloidin protection

Small discrete vacuoles in the cytoplasm of lymphocytes, sometimes overlying the nucleus, contain PAS-positive glycogen. The vacuoles are also visible in MGG preparations and are similar to those in 16.10. The majority of lymphocytes are positive in the infantile form; a smaller proportion is affected in the juvenile and adult forms. The glycogen content of the neutrophils is normal. B-lymphocytes, with their ring of PAS-positive droplets around the nucleus, should not be confused with the pathognomonic cells shown here.

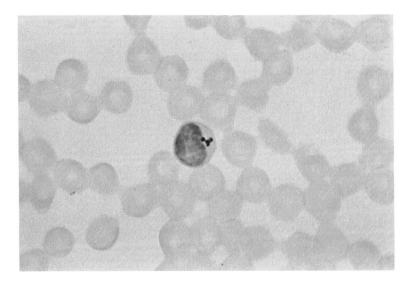

Gangliosidosis

G_{M1}-gangliosidosis type I presents in early infancy with hepatosplenomegaly, retardation, and skeletal deformities similar to those seen in the mucopolysaccharidoses. G_{M1}-gangliosidosis type II presents in the late infantile–juvenile period generally without hepatosplenomegaly or bony changes. Dementia is usual. The activity of β-galactosidase is deficient in both types. Galactosialidosis, in which sialidase is also deficient, shows the same features as type I G_{M1}-gangliosidosis.

16.20 G_{M1}-gangliosidosis type I
Blood film

Numerous vacuolated lymphocytes are present, more readily seen in the trails of the films. The vacuoles are multiple and larger than those seen in Wolman's disease or acid maltase deficiency. Similar vacuoles are found in juvenile Batten's disease, mannosidosis, infantile sialic acid storage disease, sialidosis, and I-cell disease.

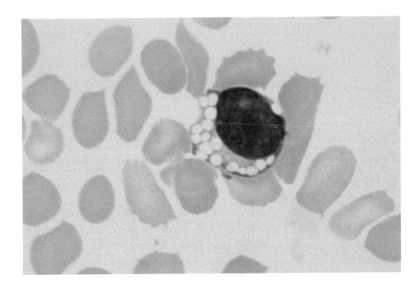

16.21 G_{M1}-gangliosidosis type I
Bone marrow

Numerous large foamy storage cells are found throughout the marrow. Lymphocytes and most other cell series also show vacuolation.

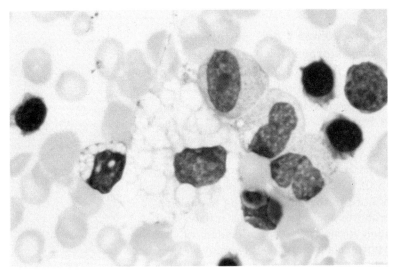

16.22 G_{M1}-gangliosidosis type I
Bone marrow

Not only are there vacuolated cells (see 16.21), but eosinophil granulocytes also have abnormal granules.

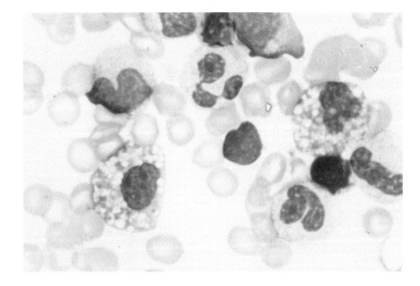

16.23 G_{M1}-gangliosidosis type II
Bone marrow

In these patients there is often no splenomegaly, but a marrow aspirate will show scattered storage cells with a 'sky-blue' cytoplasm. The cells superficially resemble Gaucher cells (see 16.3) but their characteristic blue colour distinguishes them. They also show birefringence, unlike Gaucher cells.

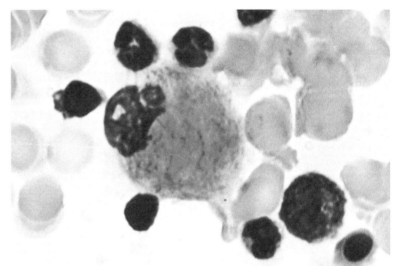

16.24 Galactosialidosis
Blood

In this disorder, the clinical presentation is similar to that of G_{M1}-gangliosidosis and deficiency of β-galactosidase is found. There is in addition deficiency of α-neuraminidase. The changes in lymphocytes and eosinophils is the same as in G_{M1}-gangliosidosis, but foamy cells may be present in a peripheral blood film, as in some cases of Wolman's disease.

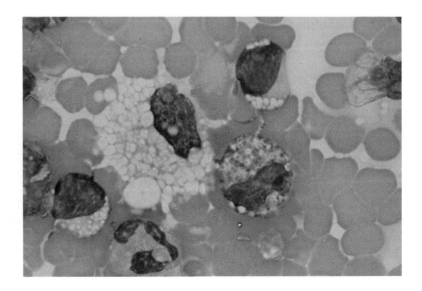

16.25   Galactosialidosis
Bone marrow

Foamy storage cells with prominent vacuoles, and storage cells containing ingested red cells and remnants of nuclear material may be seen in the marrow of this patient. The amount of ingested material is similar to that of Niemann–Pick type C (see 16.8).

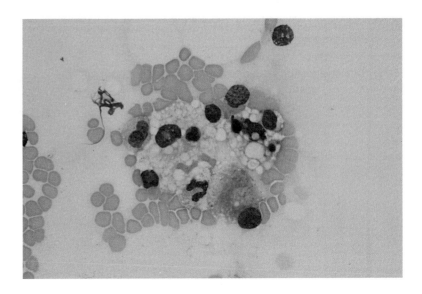

16.26   Galactosialidosis
Bone marrow

Eosinophils and eosinophil precursors show abnormal granulation similar to that seen in the peripheral blood films.

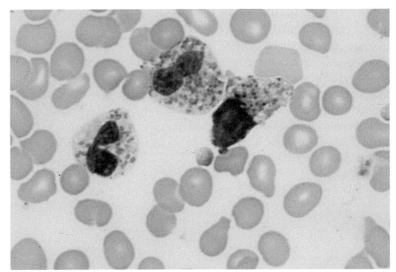

16.27   Infantile sialic acid storage disease
Blood

Numerous vacuolated lymphocytes were present in this 28-week female infant who had ascites and progressive hepatosplenomegaly. Eosinophils were very difficult to identify and where found had fewer, larger, and greyish granules (see 16.28). Free sialic acid was markedly increased in the urine. Similar but less striking vacuolation is found in the the juvenile type (Salla disease).

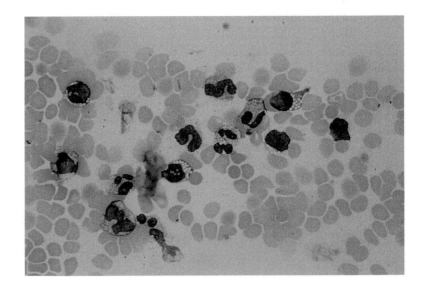

16.28 Infantile sialic acid storage disease
Blood

Eosinophils have unusual granules that are larger and fewer than normal, and stain a greyish colour. Compare the normal appearance on the left with the abnormal eosinophil on the right. Similar abnormal eosinophils are present in G_{M1}-gangliosidosis, galactosialidosis, and probably in multiple sulphatase deficiency.

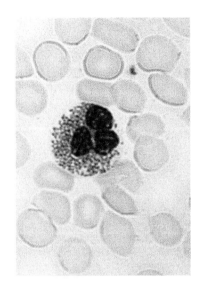
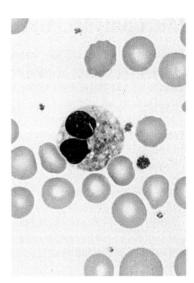

16.29 Infantile sialic acid storage disease
Bone marrow

Large foamy storage cells with large and small cytoplasmic vacuoles and some erythrophagocytosis were present in the marrow from this patient who presented in the neonatal period with a condition similar to a mucopolysaccharidosis, but without mucopolysacchariduria.

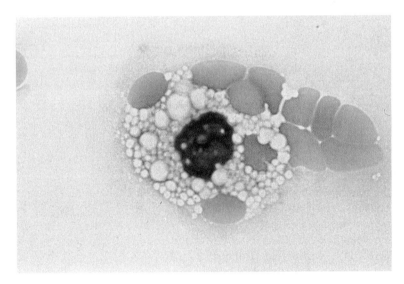

Mucopolysaccharidosis (MPS)

This group of disorders presents variably with skeletal deformities, coarse features, and hepatosplenomegaly. Mental retardation is present in most forms. Destructive behaviour is a feature of the Sanfillipo type. Urinary mucopolysaccharides (glycosaminoglycans, GAGS) are increased in all types. Table 16.1 shows the different types and their enzyme defects.

Table 16.1   The mucopolysaccharidoses

Type	Eponym	Defect
IH	Hurler	α-iduronidase
IS	Scheie	α-iduronidase
IH/S	Hurler/Scheie compound	α-iduronidase
II	Hunter (X-linked)	Sulphoiduronate sulphatase
III A	Sanfillipo	Sulphamidase
III B	,,	α-N-acetyl-glucosaminidase
III C	,,	an N-acetyl transferase
III D	,,	N-acetylglucosamine-6-sulphate sulphatase
IV A	Morquio	N-acetylgalactosamine-6-sulphate sulphatase
IV B	,,	β-galactosidase
VI	Maroteaux–Lamy	Arylsulphatase B
VII	Sly	β-glucuronidase

16.30   Mucopolysaccharidosis
Blood film; Gasser cell

These cells are lymphocytes with cytoplasmic vacuoles containing purplish granules. The purple staining represents the remnant mucopolysaccharide left after aqueous treatment. Gasser cells are present in most of the mucopolysaccharidoses except Morquio (MPS IV). Vacuolated lymphocytes are not generally a feature of the MPS and their presence will alert the observer to other diagnoses.

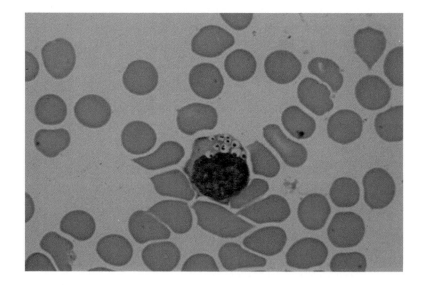

16.31 Mucopolysaccharidosis
Blood film: toluidine blue

Pink/red metachromatic granules (at the top of the cell) are present in the lymphocytes of all of the MPS except Morquio. The most prominent granulation occurs in the Sanfilippo syndrome (>20 per cent of lymphocytes affected) and in some Hunter patients. In Hurler the staining is weaker and often less than 10 per pent of lymphocytes contain metachromatic granules.

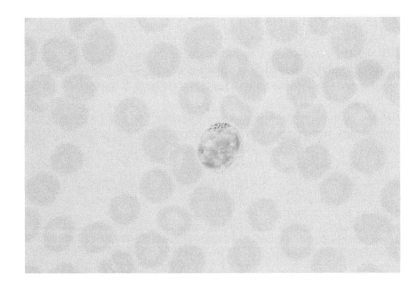

16.32 Mucopolysaccharidosis III
Bone marrow

Few storage cells are seen but the occasional large cell with stippled basophilic cytoplasm may be found. These cells will be metachromatic with toluidine blue.

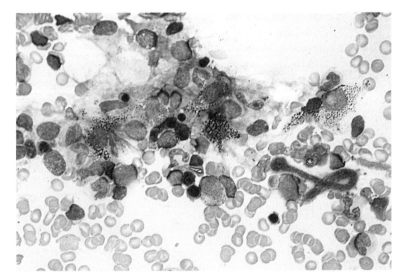

16.33 Mucopolysaccharidosis IV
Blood film

No metachromatic inclusions are present in MPS IV but within a proportion of neutrophils abnormal granulation can be found. The granules are often paired as in the figure.

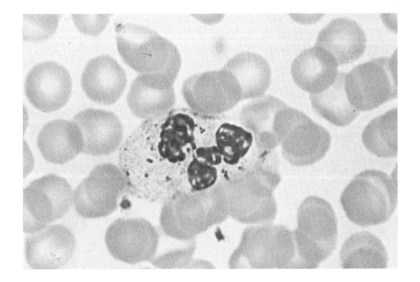

16.34   Mucopolysaccharidosis VI
Blood film; Alder granulation

All neutrophils display this rather coarse dense granulation which has some resemblance to toxic granulation. It differs in that all neutrophils are involved and in the colour which has a lilac hue. Alder granulation occurs in MPS VI (Maroteaux–Lamy), mucosulphatidosis and β-glucuronidase deficiency where it is usually much coarser. Alder granulation is also present in fetal blood in fetuses affected with these disorders, fetal blood being sampled for investigation of fetal ascites.

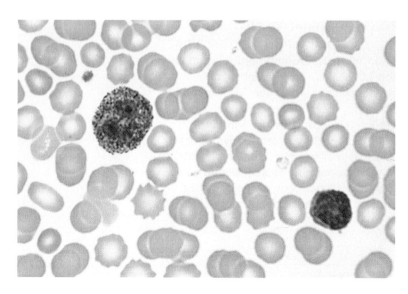

16.35   Toxic granulation
Blood film

Toxic granulation may occasionally be mistaken for Alder granulation when the staining reagents produce a more than usual redness. However, not all neutrophils are involved.

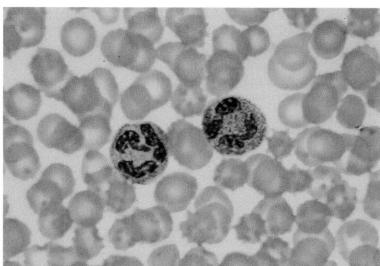

16.36   Mucopolysaccharidosis VI
Bone marrow

In MPS VI, Alder granulation is present in all granulated cells.

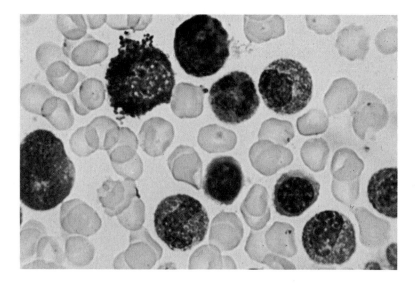

Mannosidosis

The typical presentation is of a child who appears to have one of the mucopolysaccharidoses but without mucopolysacchariduria. Deafness may be a feature. Mild forms also occur. The diagnosis can be confirmed by assay of α-mannosidase in WBC. Vacuolated lymphocytes are prominent and resemble those in G_{M1}-gangliosidosis (see 16.20), but eosinophils are normal.

16.37 Mannosidosis
Bone marrow
Numerous foamy storage cells are present. The vacuoles are mainly small. The storage material is very water soluble and is not stained by conventional methods.

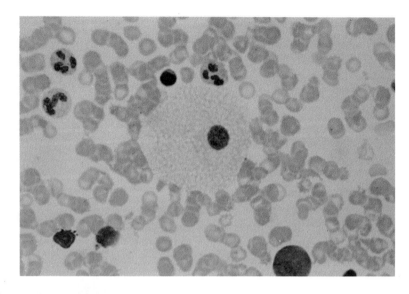

16.38 Mannosidosis
Bone marrow
Scattered plasma cells with striking vacuolation are present. The vacuoles are separated by strands of blue-staining cytoplasm. These cells are present in mannosidosis and fucosidosis.

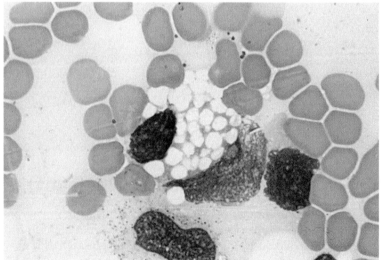

16.39   Fucosidosis
Bone marrow

Foamy storage cells, some showing marked haemophagocytosis, others with gross vacuolation, are seen. Many of the cells are strongly PAS-positive. Patients with fucosidosis present similarly to those with the mucopolysaccharidoses, but without mucopolysacchariduria. Some have angiokeratomata.

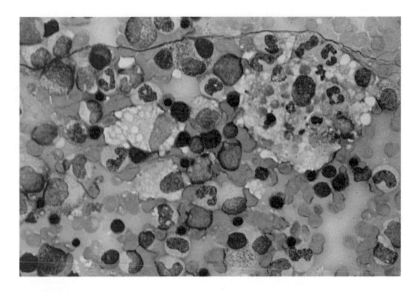

16.40   Fucosidosis
Bone marrow

Plasma cells, similar to those in mannosidosis, can be seen.

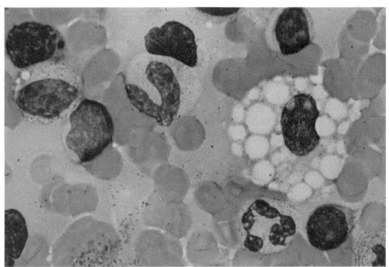

Sialidosis (neuraminidase deficiency)

Sialidosis I, also known as the cherry-red spot myoclonus syndrome, presents in the juvenile period and has no visceromegaly. Lymphocyte morphology is normal. Sialidosis II, formerly known as mucolipidosis I presents as a mucopolysaccharidosis without mucopolysacchariduria. The lymphocytes are vacuolated and are very similar to those of juvenile Batten's disease and G_{M1}-gangliosidosis (see 16.20).

16.41 Sialidosis I
Bone marrow
Storage cells with large bluish staining vacuoles can be found with some difficulty. They resemble odd plasma cells.

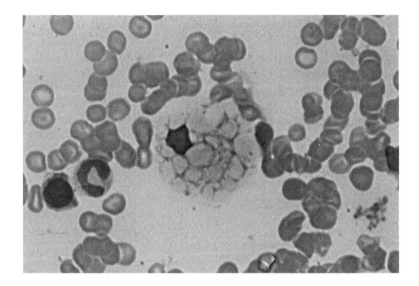

16.42 Sialidosis I
Bone marrow; PAS
The storage cells are intensely stained and are unlike any other storage cell.

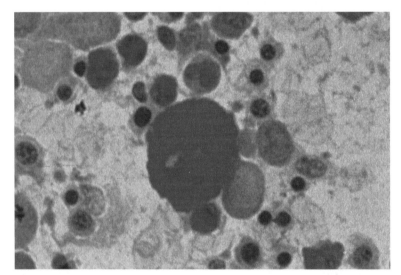

16.43 Sialidosis I
Bone marrow; acid phosphatase (Gömöri) reaction
The storage cells are strongly reactive at the periphery of the vacuoles. The activity of the other cells present is punctate and normal.

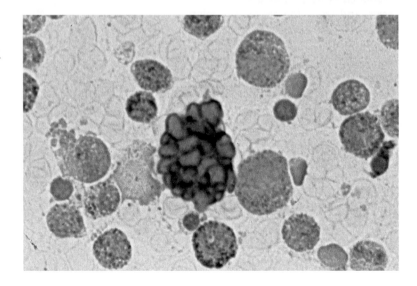

16.44　I-cell disease (Mucolipidosis II)
Bone marrow

Patients with I-cell disease present as a mucopolysaccharidosis without mucopolysacchariduria and are usually of very short stature. Contractures and cardiac involvement occur in the second year. The bone marrow generally shows little of note except for occasional vacuolated osteoblasts with pinkish inclusions. Peripheral lymphocytes are vacuolated and like those in G_{M1}-gangliosidosis (see 16.20).

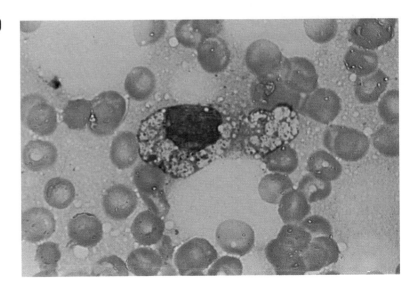

Batten's disease

This group of disorders occurs in four main types, each with different clinical and pathological features. The **infantile** form presents with psychomotor retardation from about 8 months. Microcephaly and an isoelectric EEG are later features. No abnormality of blood cells is seen by light microscopy. The **late infantile** form presents with slowing of development and severe seizures and dementia from around 18 months to 3 years. The EEG changes are characteristic. No abnormality of blood cells is found by light microscopy. The **juvenile** form presents from 5-8 years with progressive loss of vision, followed by dementia sometimes several years later. Vacuolated lymphocytes are always present. The **early juvenile** form (sometimes referred to as the variant late infantile form) presents around 4 years with ataxia and dementia with a more rapid progess the the juvenile form. The EEG is as for the late infantile type. No changes are found in blood cells by light or electron microscopy.

16.45　Juvenile Batten's disease
Blood

Vacuolated lymphocytes are always present and show the coarse vacuolation seen here. These appearances are the same as those in G_{M1}-gangliosidosis, mannosidosis, and sialic acid storage disease and diagnosis will depend on the clinical history. Electron microscopy usually adds nothing more.

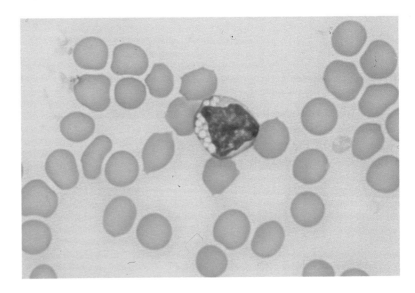

16.46 Late infantile Batten's disease
Buffy coat preparation for electron microscopy

The curvilinear bodies, pathognomonic of late infantile Batten's disease are present in lymphocytes. They occur in more than 10% of lymphocytes.

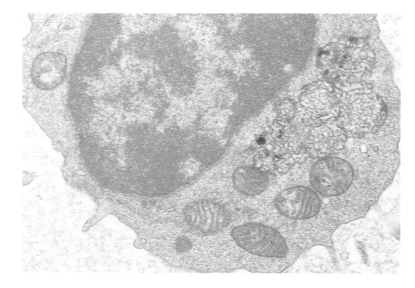

16.47 Infantile Batten's disease
Buffy coat preparation for electron microscopy

The granular osmiophilic deposits (GROD) are found in about 10 per cent of lymphocytes. The inclusions must be distinguished from the normally occurring parallel tubular arrays, and from the tubuloreticular structures found in immune mediated disorders. The clinical context of the request is as always important.

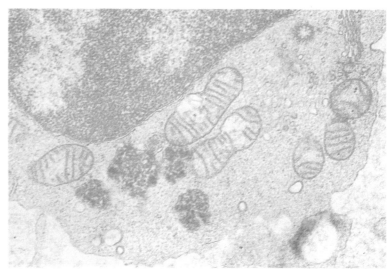

Cystinosis

Failure to thrive and a Fanconi syndrome are the presenting features. Photophobia and fair hair are also common. Diagnosis is now mainly by biochemical assay of the cystine content of WBC. Although cystine crystals have been reported in WBC, they are sufficiently rare for there to be no examples to illustrate.

16.48   Cystinosis
Bone marrow; alcoholic basic fuchsin

The storage cells containing the cystine crystals are fragile and the films must be made carefully, and stained in an alcoholic solution to retain the water-soluble cystine. Films are best viewed in partially polarized light. The brick shaped crystals are pathognomonic, as are the hexagonal (end-on) forms.

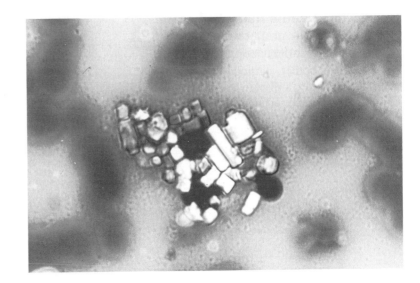

16.49   Cystinosis
Bone marrow; wet preparation

A single drop from the anticoagulated sample is placed on a microscope slide, covered by a cover slip and viewed in polarized light. The hexagonal habit is not birefringent, but the brick shaped crystals are.

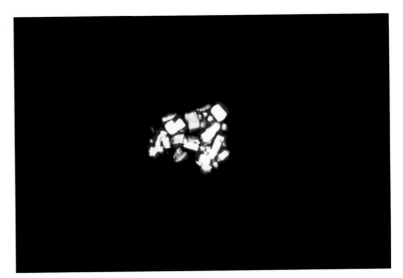

16.50   Oxalosis
Bone marrow trephine; polarized light

Oxalate crystals with their characteristic fan shape are present in the bone, but not in the marrow cavity.

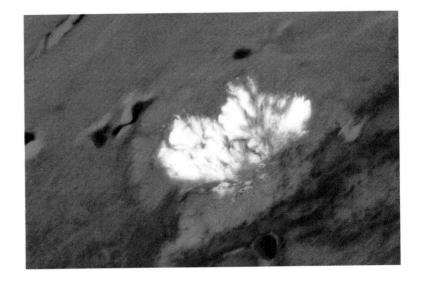

16.51   Jordans anomaly
Blood

Neutrophils show prominent vacuolation, which is also present in eosinophils, basophils, and monocytes but not in lymphocytes.

Jordans' patients had a muscular disorder which could have been a fat oxidation defect or more probably had neutral lipid storage disease. This disorder has ichthyosis as a prominent feature and all patients with ichthyosis should have a blood film examined.

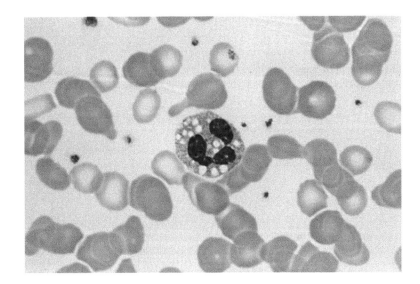

16.52   Jordans anomaly
Blood; Oil Red O for neutral fat

The prominently vacuolated neutrophils (and other vacuolated cells) contain neutral fat. No toxic granulation is present.

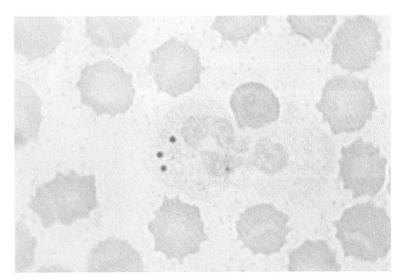

16.53   Hyperlipoproteinaemia type I
Bone marrow

Acquired storage cells filled with lipid, accumulate in response to the lipid overload and may be mistaken for storage cells. This patient presented with anaemia and splenomegaly. The anaemia was treated but the spleen continued to enlarge. The bone-marrow aspirate revealed these cells which were interpreted as Niemann–Pick cells, and it was not until the very lipaemic serum was discovered that the diagnosis was made. A low-fat diet resulted in a smaller spleen.

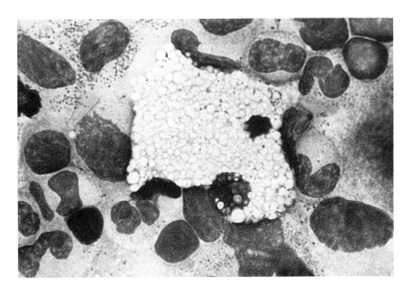

16.54   Fetal G$_{M1}$-gangliosidosis type I
Blood

Vacuolated lymphocytes were present in an affected 18-week fetus.

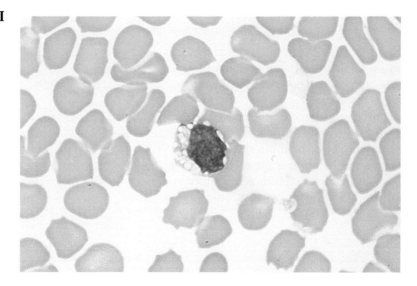

16.55   Fetal mucopolysaccharidosis VI
Bone marrow

The storage cells are present in fetal marrow from at least 11 weeks' gestation. The examination of a marrow sample provides the quickest verification of an affected fetus after biochemical detection of the disease in a chorionic villus sample. Storage cells are found in the fetal marrow in all visceral storage disorders.

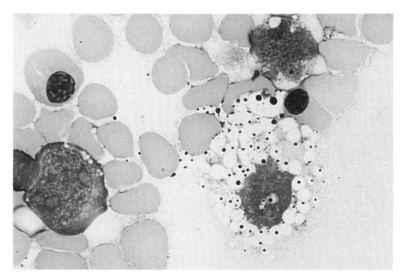

16.56   Actin storage disease (Brandalise syndrome) (Ribeiro et al. (1994). *Blood*, **83**, 3717)
Bone marrow

Bright blue inclusions were present in about 30 per cent of myeloid cells and in occasional monocytes, megakaryocytes, lymphocytes, and neutrophils in the bone-marrow aspirate. The sample came from a 13-month-old boy with transfusion dependent anaemia, splenomegaly, and striking grey skin discoloration. He also had intermittent neutropenia, abnormal neutrophil migration, and abnormal platelet aggregation. The anaemia and grey skin discolouration resolved spontaneously but the inclusions persisted. Immunocytochemistry showed the inclusions contained muscle-specific actin.

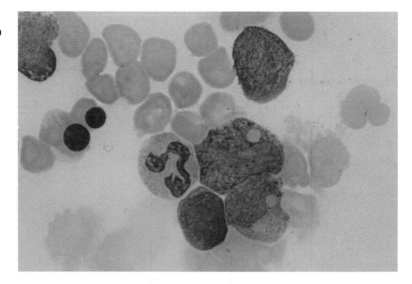

16.57 Actin storage disease (Brandalise syndrome)
Blood

The bright blue inclusions were present in neutrophils and lymphocytes from the same patient as in 16.56. Similar inclusions have been seen transiently in a variety of situations with no particular clinical setting. The transient inclusions have usually disappeared within a month, unlike those in actin storage disease.

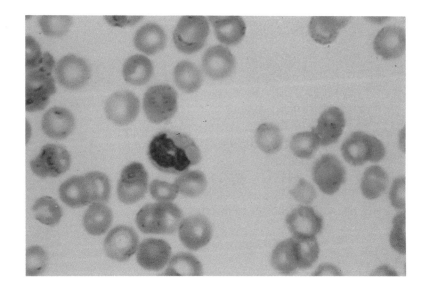

17
Artefacts

17.1 Red cell crenation
Blood film

This effect is caused by rapid drying of the blood film on a hot day. These are echinocytes and not acanthocytes.

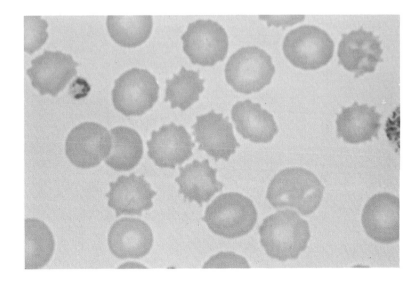

17.2 Sequestrene change
Blood film

Prolonged exposure of blood samples to sequestrene often leads to nuclear condensation in polymorphs. Lymphocytes are more resistant. This change may also be seen in viraemia and septicaemia.

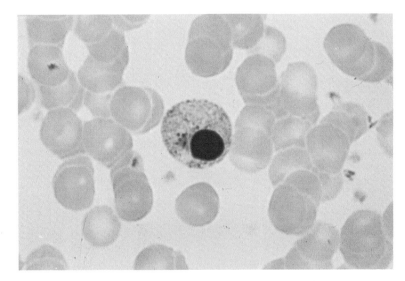

17.3   Sequestrene change
Blood film

Red cell crenation and neutrophil nuclear disintegration have occurred after sustained exposure to sequestrene.

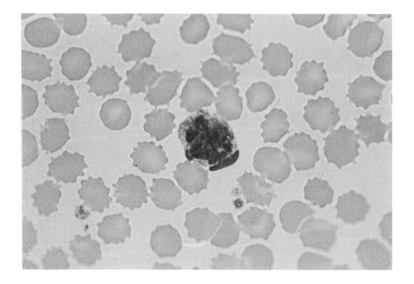

17.4   Water artefact
Blood film

Substantial water contamination of the methanol fixative will produce small red cell inclusions.

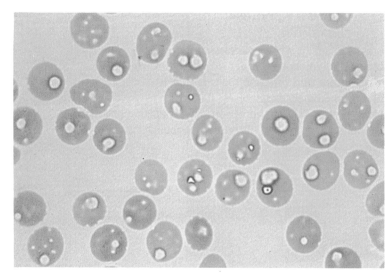

17.5   Water artefact
Blood film

In this instance, because of the high concentration of water, the inclusions have fused to form large vacuoles superficially mimicking gross hypochromia.

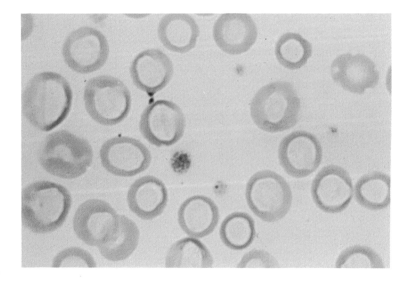

17.6   Auto-agglutination of red cells
Blood film

This child had mycoplasma pneumonia.
The red cells have auto-agglutinated
because they are coated with cold
antibody. This agglutination occurs as the
slide is dried at room temperature, and
can be prevented by drying at 37 °C.

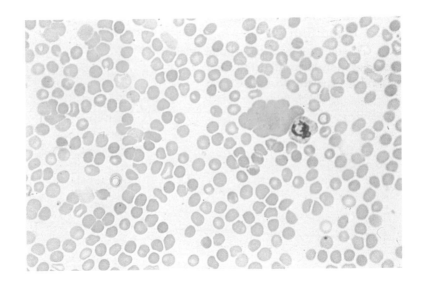

17.7   Platelet satellitism
Blood film

This artefact in which platelets 'rosette'
around polymorphs, occurs at room
temperature and in some cases is due to
an IgG-mediated mechanism. Lack of
awareness of this phenomenon may lead
to a false diagnosis of thrombocytopenia.

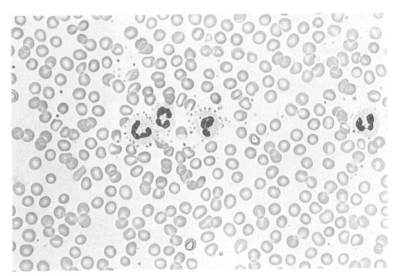

17.8   Platelet aggregation
Blood film

This effect may be seen in films made after
a difficult thumb-prick procedure and
must be differentiated from true
thrombocytopenia.

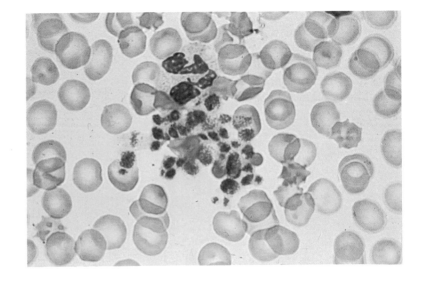

17.9 EDTA-mediated platelet clumping
Blood film

This phenomenon, due to an IgG antibody coating the platelets, causes clumping in the presence of EDTA but not other anticoagulants. It is thus another cause of 'pseudo-thrombocytopenia'.

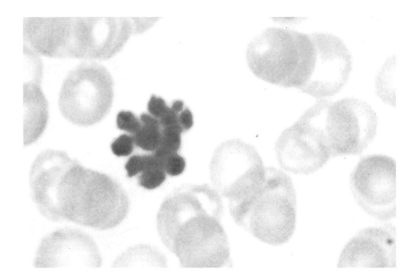

17.10 'Talc' granules
Bone marrow

Starch granules, now used instead of talc, can mimic storage cells, parasites, or even cryptosporidia. The granules, which get on to the slides from surgical gloves, are brightly PAS-positive and have a maltese cross birefringence.

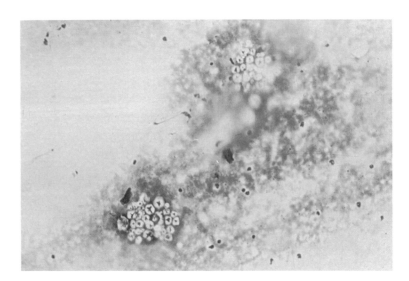

17.11 'Pseudo-rosette'
Bone marrow

Poor spreading of marrow aspirates may lead to artificial clumps or 'rosettes', mimicking tumour infiltration, e.g. neuroblastoma.

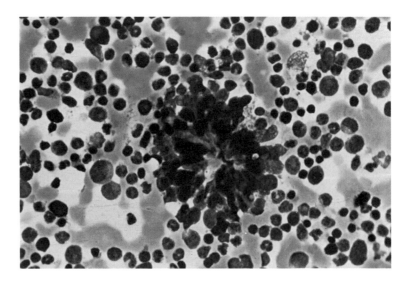

17.12   Triglyceride crystals
Bone marrow, polarized light

On exposure to air, the triglyceride (fat) present in most marrow samples crystallizes, in unfixed marrow films, to form the needle-shaped crystals shown here. Triglyceride is removed by fixation in methanol and crystals are not seen in fixed films. The crystals could be mistaken for tyrosine, uric acid, various phosphates, or drug metabolites.

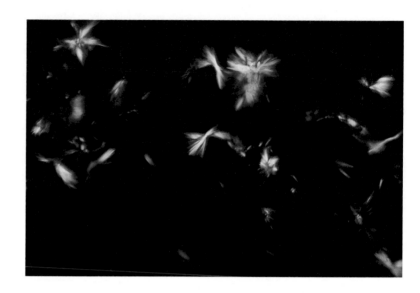

17.13   Cocci in neutrophil
Blood

This sample was taken by fingerprick from an area of skin heavily contaminated with staphylococci. The neutrophil has phagocytosed them *in vitro*. The intact nature of the cocci probably indicates a very recent event and is a feature only rarely seen in septicaemia.

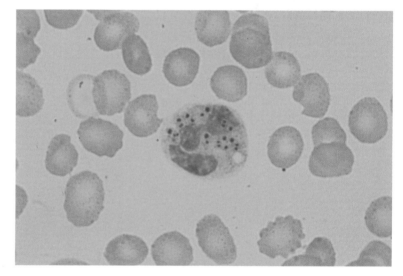

18
Reference values

Contents

Table 18.1   Normal blood count values in childhood

Age	Hb (g/dl)	RBC (×10¹²/l)	Haematocrit	MCV (fl)	WBC (×10⁹/l)	Neutrophils (×10⁹/l)	Lymphocytes (×10⁹/l)	Monocytes (×10⁹/l)	Eosinophils (×10⁹/l)	Platelets (×10⁹/l)
Birth	14.9–23.7	3.7–6.5	0.47–0.75	100–135	10.0–26.0	2.7–14.4	2.0–7.3	0–1.9	0–0.84	
2 weeks	13.4–19.8	3.9–5.9	0.41–0.65	88–120	6.0–21.0	1.8–5.4	2.8–9.1	0.1–1.7	0–0.84	
2 months	9.4–13.0	3.1–4.3	0.28–0.42	84–105	6.0–18.0	1.2–7.5	3.0–13.5	0.1–1.7	0.1–0.8	150–450
6 months	11.1–14.1	3.9–5.5	0.31–0.41	68–82	6.0–17.5	1.0–8.5	4.0–13.5	0.2–1.2	0.3–0.8	at all
1 year	11.3–14.1	4.1–5.3	0.33–0.41	71–85	6.0–17.5	1.5–8.5	4.0–10.5	0.2–1.2	0.3–0.8	ages
2–6 years	11.5–13.5	3.9–5.3	0.34–0.40	75–87	5.0–17.0	1.5–8.5	1.5–9.5	0.2–1.2	0.3–0.8	
6–12 years	11.5–15.5	4.0–5.2	0.35–0.45	77–95	4.5–14.5	1.5–8.0	1.5–7.0	0.2–1.0	0.1–0.5	
12–18 years										
Female	12.0–16.0	4.1–5.1	0.36–0.46	78–95	4.5–13.0	1.8–8.0	1.2–6.5	0.2–0.8	<0.1–0.5	
Male	13.0–16.0	4.5–5.3	0.37–0.49	78–95						

Data given as approximate ranges, compiled from various sources.
Red cell values at birth derived from skin puncture blood; most other data from venous blood.
Reproduced from Hinchliffe (1992) by permission of Churchill Livingstone.

Table 18.2   Red cell values (mean ± 1 SD) on the first postnatal day from 24 weeks' gestational age

Gestational age (weeks) (No of infants)	24–25 (n = 7)	26–27 (n = 11)	28–29 (n = 7)	30–31 (n = 35)	32–33 (n = 23)	34–35 (n = 23)	36–37 (n = 20)	Term (n = 19)
RBC (×10¹²/l)	4.65 ± 0.43	4.73 ± 0.45	4.62 ± 0.75	4.79 ± 0.74	5.0 ± 0.76	5.09 ± 0.5	5.27 ± 0.68	5.14 ± 0.7
Hb (g/dl)	19.4 ± 1.5	19.0 ± 2.5	19.3 ± 1.8	19.1 ± 2.2	18.5 ± 2.0	19.6 ± 2.1	19.2 ± 1.7	19.3 ± 2.2
Haematocrit	0.63 ± 0.04	0.62 ± 0.08	0.60 ± 0.07	0.60 ± 0.08	0.60 ± 0.08	0.61 ± 0.07	0.64 ± 0.07	0.61 ± 0.074
MCV (fl)	135 ± 0.2	132 ± 14.4	131 ± 13.5	127 ± 12.7	123 ± 15.7	122 ± 10.0	121 ± 12.5	119 ± 9.4
Reticulocytes (%)	6.0 ± 0.5	9.6 ± 3.2	7.5 ± 2.5	5.8 ± 2.0	5.0 ± 1.9	3.9 ± 1.6	4.2 ± 1.8	3.2 ± 1.4
Weight (g)	725 ± 185	993 ± 194	1174 ± 128	1450 ± 232	1816 ± 192	1957 ± 291	2245 ± 213	

Counts performed on skin puncture blood.
Reproduced from Zaizov and Matoth (1976), by permission of Alan R. Liss Inc.

Table 18.3   Mean haematological values in the first 2 weeks of life in the term infant

Haematological value	Cord blood	Day 1	Day 3	Day 7	Day 14
Hb (g/dl)	16.8	18.4	17.8	17.0	16.8
Haematocrit	0.53	0.58	0.55	0.54	0.52
Red cells (×10¹²/l)	5.25	5.8	5.6	5.2	5.1
MCV (fl)	107	108	99.0	98.0	96.0
MCH (pg)	34	35	33	32.5	31.5
MCHC (%)	31.7	32.5	33	33	33
Reticulocytes (%)	3–7	3–7	1–3	0–1	0–1
Nucleated RBC (mm³)	500	200	0–5	0	0
Platelets (×10⁹/l)	290	192	213	248	252

Reproduced from Oski (1982), by permission of Dr F. Oski and W. B. Saunders Co.

Table 18.4 Haemoglobin (Hb), haematocrit (Hct), and red blood cell (RBC) counts in term African neonates

	Number tested	Hb	Mean ± 1 SD Hct	RBC
Day 1	304	15.6 ± 2.0	0.450 ± 0.065	4.00 ± 0.67
3	261	15.5 ± 2.1	0.442 ± 0.062	3.91 ± 0.61
7	249	14.2 ± 2.3	0.413 ± 0.063	3.67 ± 0.55
Week 2	233	13.1 ± 1.9	0.391 ± 0.043	3.45 ± 0.56
3	145	11.7 ± 1.8	0.356 ± 0.050	3.27 ± 0.47
4	117	10.6 ± 1.6	0.325 ± 0.044	3.01 ± 0.48

Values are lower than those reported in neonates from Europe and North America. Summarized from Scott–Emuakpor et al. (1985a).

Table 18.5 Haemoglobin values (median and 95% range) in the first 6 months of life in iron–sufficient (serum ferritin $\geqslant 10$ µg/l) preterm infants

Age	Birth weight (g) 1000–1500	Number tested	Birth weight (g) 1501–2000	Number tested
2 weeks	16.3 (11.7–18.4)	17	14.8 (11.8–19.6)	39
1 month	10.9 (8.7–15.2)	15	11.5 (8.2–15.0)	42
2 months	8.8 (7.1–11.5)	17	9.4 (8.0–11.4)	47
3 months	9.8 (8.9–11.2)	16	10.2 (9.3–11.8)	41
4 months	11.3 (9.1–13.1)	13	11.3 (9.1–13.1)	37
5 months	11.6 (10.2–14.3)	8	11.8 (10.4–13.0)	21
6 months	12.0 (9.4–13.8)	9	11.8 (10.7–12.6)	21

All had an uncomplicated course in the first 2 weeks of life and none received exchange transfusion.
Counts obtained from venous and skin–puncture blood.
Reproduced from Lundstrom et al. (1977) by permission of Dr. M. A. Siimes and the C. V. Mosby Co.

Table 18.6 Normal values for Hb, RBC, and RBC indices in the first year of life

Hb/RBC value	0.5 (n = 232)	1 (n = 240)	2 (n = 241)	Age (months) 4 (n = 52)	6 (n = 52)	9 (n = 56)	12 (n = 56)
Hb (g/dl)	16.6	13.9	11.2	12.2	12.6	12.7	12.7
−2 SD	13.4	10.7	9.4	10.3	11.1	11.4	11.3
Hct	0.53	0.44	0.35	0.38	0.36	0.36	0.37
−2 SD	0.41	0.33	0.28	0.32	0.31	0.32	0.33
RBC ($\times 10^{12}$/l)	4.9	4.3	3.7	4.3	4.7	4.7	4.7
−2 SD, +2 SD	3.9–5.9	3.3–5.3	3.1–4.3	3.5–5.1	3.9–5.5	4.0–5.3	4.1–5.3
MCH (pg)	33.6	32.5	30.4	28.6	26.8	27.3	26.8
−2 SD	30	29	27	25	24	25	24
MCV (fl)	105.3	101.3	94.8	86.7	76.3	77.7	77.7
−2 SD	88	91	84	76	68	70	71
MCHC %	31.4	31.8	31.8	32.7	35.0	34.9	34.3
−2 SD	28.1	28.1	28.3	28.8	32.7	32.4	32.1

Values after the age of 2 months were obtained from an iron-supplemented group in whom iron deficiency was excluded.
Counts performed on venous blood. Values given are mean and standard deviation (SD).
Reproduced from Saarinen and Siimes (1978), by permission of the Dr M. A. Siimes and C. V. Mosby Co.

Fig. 18.1 Hb, MCHC, RBC, and MCV (mean ± 1 SD) values in Jamaican children aged from one day to 5 years. A cohort of 243 children was studied, although the data at each point are derived from varying numbers. Regular iron and folate supplements were not given. ● = boys, ○ = girls. Reproduced from Serjeant *et al.* (1980) by permission of Blackwell Scientific Publications.

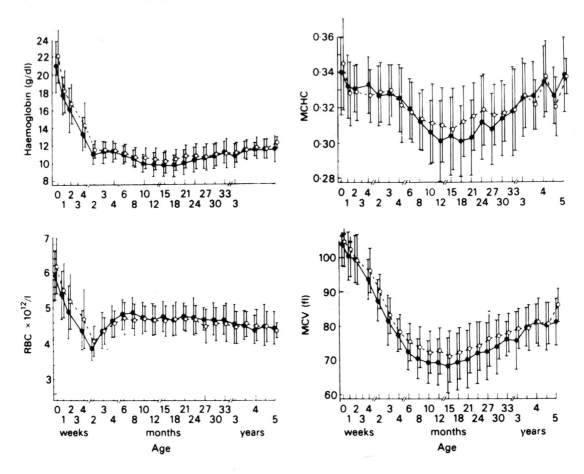

Table 18.7 Reticulocyte count (percentage and absolute counts mean ± 2 SD) in children. Summarized from Böck and Herkner (1994)

Age	n	Percentage	Absolute count (10^9/l)
Term newborns	150	2.4 ± 2.30	74.2 ± 50.0
Preterm newborns	30	2.55 ± 2.02	71.8 ± 57.6
1 week–16 years	750	1.16 ± 0.78	58.7 ± 24.6

Fig. 18.2 Hb and MCV percentiles for girls and boys derived from non–indigent white children in California and Finland. Hb values obtained from 9946 children, MCV values from 2314; none had laboratory evidence of iron deficiency or haemoglobinopathy. Reproduced from Dallman and Siimes (1979) by permission of the C. V. Mosby Co.

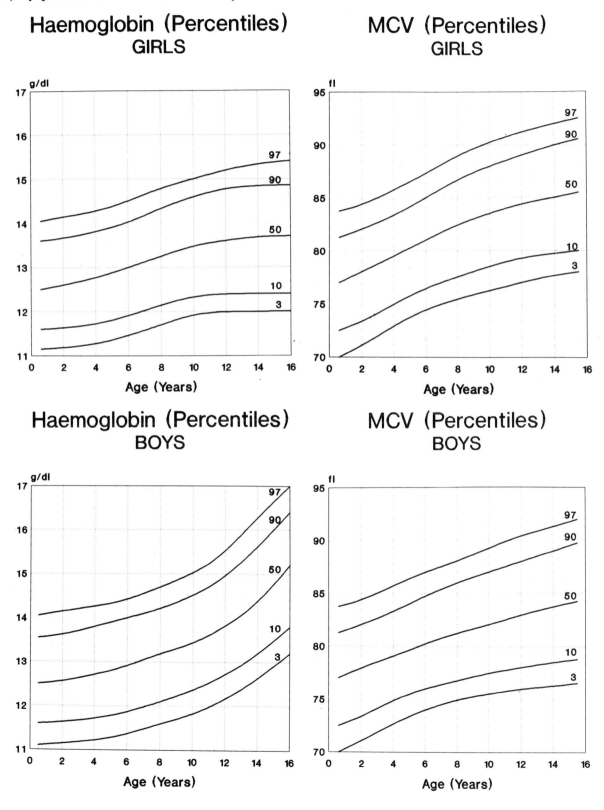

Table 18.8   Differential leukocyte values ($\times 10^9$/l) in 1216 children 0–16 years old. The ranges given are based on mean $\pm$ 2 SD after logarithmic transformation whenever necessary

Parameter	Age in years																	
	8 days	0	1	2	3	4	5	6	7	8	9	10	11	12	13	14	15	16
Neutrophils	2.1–8.0	1.5–6.9				1.8–7.7		1.5–5.9									1.7–5.7	
Lymphocytes	3.3–9.4	3.5–10.0	2.6–9.3	2.3–8.4	1.8–6.0		1.7–4.6		1.5–4.1									
Monocytes	0.03–0.98	0.21–1.64	0.15–1.28															
Eosinophils	0.16–0.94	0.06–0.62		0.04–1.19		0.09–1.04		0.08–1.01				0.04–0.76						
Basophils	0.02–0.12																	

Summarised from Cranendonk *et al.* (1985).

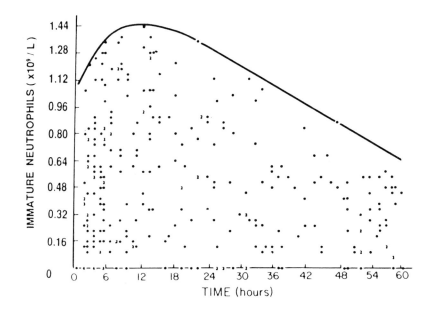

Fig. 18.3   Total neutrophil count ($\times 10^9$/l; including band cells and earlier forms) in the first 60 hours of life. Each dot represents a single value and numbers represent the number of values at the same point. Data based on automated leucocyte count and 100–cell differential. Reproduced from Manroe *et al.* (1979) by permission of the C. V. Mosby Co.

Fig. 18.4   Reference range for immature neutrophils ($\times 10^9$/l) in the first 60 hours of life. Data obtained and expressed as in Fig. 18.3. Reproduced from Manroe *et al.* (1979) by permission of the C. V. Mosby Co.

Table 18.9   Values for mature and immature neutrophils and the immature/total neutrophil ratio in 24 infants of < 33 weeks' gestation

Age (hrs)	Mature neutrophils ($\times$ 10^9/l) Median (range)	Immature neutrophils ($\times$ 10^9/l) Median (range)	Immature/total ratio Median (range)
1	4.64	0.11	0.04
(n = 10)	(2.20–8.18)	(0–1.5)	(0–0.35)
12	6.80	0.27	0.04
(n = 17)	(4.0–22.48)	(0–1.6)	(0–0.21)
24	5.60	0.14	0.03
(n = 17)	(2.61–21.20)	(0–3.66)	(0–0.17)
48	4.98	0.13	0.02
(n = 20)	(1.02–14.43)	(0–2.15)	(0–0.17)
72	3.19	0.16	0.3
(n = 22)	(1.28–13.94)	(0–2.42)	(0–0.25)
96	3.44	0.23	0.05
(n = 21)	(1.37–16.56)	(0–3.95)	(0–0.37)
120	3.46	0.25	0.05
(n = 17)	(1.27–15.00)	(0–2.89)	(0–0.21)

Summarised from Lloyd and Oto (1982).

Table 18.10   Normal limits of the immature/total and immature/segmented granulocyte ratios in healthy neonates

	Day 1	Day 7	Day 28	Reference
Immature/total	0.16	0.12	0.12	Manroe *et al.* (1979)
Immature/total (African)	0.22	0.21	0.18	Scott-Emuakpor *et al.* (1985*b*)
Immature/segmented	0.3	0.3	0.3	Zipursky and Jaber (1978)

Reproduced from Hinchliffe and Lilleyman (1987), by permission of John Wiley and Sons Ltd.

Fig. 18.5 Neutrophil count ($\times 10^9$/l; bar indicates ± 1 SD) during the first 14 days of life in babies of appropriate weight for gestational age (●) and babies who were small for gestational age (○). Reproduced from McIntosh *et al.* (1988) by permission of Professor N. McIntosh and the Editor of *Archives of Disease in Childhood.*

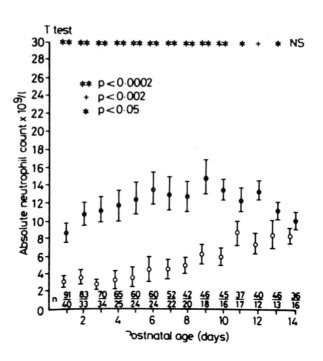

Table 18.11 Numbers ($\times 10^9$/l; mean 1 SD) of CD3 (T cell) CD4 (helper/inducer T cell) CD8 (suppressor/cytotoxic T cell) and CD20 (B cell) lymphocytes in peripheral blood of children. Summarized from Panaro *et al.* (1991).

Age	Number	CD3	CD4	CD8	CD20
1–3 days	18	4.36 ± 1.22	3.31 ± 1.01	1.31 ± 0.46	1.01 ± 0.46
<6 months	23	3.64 ± 1.66	2.38 ± 0.87	1.07 ± 0.52	2.04 ± 0.89
>−12 months	15	3.52 ± 0.99	2.31 ± 0.67	1.14 ± 0.36	1.79 ± 0.63
1–2 years	20	3.39 ± 1.11	1.88 ± 0.48	0.99 ± 0.19	1.59 ± 0.52
3–5 years	18	3.03 ± 0.92	1.51 ± 0.59	1.23 ± 0.42	1.02 ± 0.60
6–10 years	23	2.28 ± 0.91	1.08 ± 0.40	0.90 ± 0.40	0.50 ± 0.23
11–17 years (male)	23	2.12 ± 0.70	1.13 ± 0.45	0.88 ± 0.40	0.52 ± 0.23

Table 18.12 Mean and range of values for neutrophils, band forms, and lymphocytes ($\times 10^9$/l) in African neonates[1]

	Day 1	Day 7	Day 28
Neutrophils	5.67 (0.98–12.9)	2.01 (0.57–6.5)	1.67 (0.65–3.2)
Band forms	1.16 (0.16–2.3)	0.55 (0–1.5)	0.36 (0–0.39)
Lymphocytes	5.10 (1.4–8.0)	5.63 (2.2–15.5)	0.55 (3.2–9.9)

[1]Data based on 100-cell differential count.
The lower range of neutrophil values known to occur in negroes is evident in the neonatal period. Summarized from Scott-Emuakpor *et al.* (1985*b*); reproduced from Hinchliffe and Lilleyman (1987), by permission of John Wiley and Sons Ltd.

Fig. 18.6
Platelet count ($\times 10^9$/l; bar indicates
± 1 SD) during the first 14 days of life in
babies of appropriate weight for
gestational age (●) and babies who were
small for gestational age (○). Reproduced
from McIntosh *et al.* (1988) by permission
of Professor N. McIntosh and the Editor
of *Archives of Disease in Childhood.*

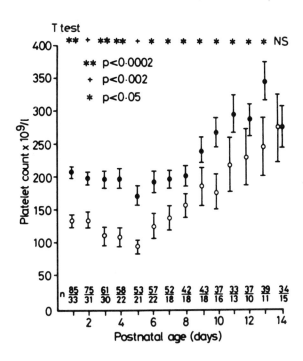

Table 18.13 Normal progenitor cell numbers during development

Age	PB BFU-E	PB CFU-GM	PB CFU-Meg
Fetuses 18–20 weeks	75–1500	20–700	1–10
Birth, term	40–100	10–200	5–20
Adults	5–40	5–20	2–10

Data shown are approximate ranges derived from various sources, and indicate
numbers of progenitor cells per 10^5 mononuclear cells plated.
Abbreviations: PB = peripheral blood; BFU-E = burst-forming-unit-erythroid; CFU-
GM = colony-forming-unit-granulocyte-macrophage; CFU-Meg = colony-forming-
unit-megakaryocyte
Summarized from Auerbach and Alter (1989).

References

Auerbach, A. D. and Alter B. P. (1989). Prenatal and postnatal diagnosis of aplastic anaemia. In: Alter B. P. (ed) Perinatal Hematology. *Methods in Haematology*, **19**, 225–51. Churchill Livingstone, Edinburgh.

Böck, A. and Herkner K. R. (1994). Reticulocyte maturity pattern analysis as a predictive marker of erythropoiesis in paediatrics. Part I: evaluation of age-dependent reference values. *Clinical and Laboratory Haematology*, **16**, 247–51.

Cranendonk, E., van Gennip A. H., Abeling N. G. G. M., Behrendt, H., and Hast, A. A. M. (1985). Reference values for automated cytochemical differential count of leukocytes in children 0–16 years old: comparison with manually obtained counts from Wright-stained smears. *Journal of Clinical Chemistry and Clinical Biochemistry*, **23**, 663–7.

Dallman, P. R. and Siimes, M. A. (1979). Percentile curves for haemoglobin and red cell volume in infancy and childhood. *Journal of Pediatrics*, **94**, 26–31.

Hinchliffe, R. F. and Lilleyman J. S. (eds) (1987). *Practical paediatric haematology*. John Wiley and Sons, Chichester.

Lloyd, B. W. and Oto, A. (1982). Normal values for mature and immature neutrophils in very preterm babies. *Archives of Disease in Childhood*, **57**, 233–5.

Lundstrom, U., Siimes, M. A., and Dallman, P. R. (1977). At what age does iron supplementation become necessary in low birthweight infants? *Journal of Pediatrics*, **91**, 878–83.

McIntosh, N., Kempson, C., and Tyler, R. M. (1988). Blood counts in extremely low birthweight infants. *Archives of Disease in Childhood*, **63**, 74–6.

Manroe, B. L., Weinberg, A. G., Rosenfeld, C. R., and Browne, R. (1979). The neonatal blood count in health and disease. 1. Reference values for neutrophilic cells. *Journal of Pediatrics*, **95**, 89–98.

Oski, F. A. (1982). Normal blood values in the newborn period. In: *Hematologic problems in the newborn*, (ed. F. A. Oski and J. L. Naiman), pp. 1–31. W. B. Saunders, Philadelphia.

Panaro, A., Amati, A., di Loreto, M., Felle, R., Ferrante M., Papadia, A. M., *et al.* (1991). Lymphocyte subpopulations in pediatric age. Definition of reference values by flow cytometry. *Allergologia et Immunopathologia*, **19**, 109–12.

Saarinen, U. M. and Siimes, M. A. (1978). Developmental changes in red blood cell counts and indices of infants after exclusion of iron deficiency by laboratory criteria and continuous iron supplementation. *Journal of Pediatrics*, **92**, 412–16.

Scott-Emuakpor, A. B., Okolo, A. A., Omene, J. A., and Ukpe, S. I. (1985a). Normal haematological values of the African neonate. *Blut*, **51**, 11–18.

Scott-Emuakpor, A. B., Okolo, A. A., Omene, J. A., and Ukpe, S. I. (1985b). Pattern of leucocytes in blood of healthy African neonates. *Acta Haematologica*, **74**, 104–7.

Serjeant, G. R., Grandison, Y., Mason, K., Serjeant, B., Sewell, A., and Vaidya, S. (1980). Haematological indices in normal negro children : a Jamaican cohort from birth to five years. *Clinical and Laboratory Haematology*, **2**, 169–178.

Zaizov, R. and Matoth, Y. (1976). Red cell values on the first postnatal day during the last 16 weeks of gestation. *American Journal of Hematology*, **1**, 272–78.

Zipursky, A. and Jaber, H. M. (1978). The haematology of bacterial infection in newborn infants. *Clinics in Haematology*, **7**, 175–93.

Index